The Type 2 Diabetes Sourcebook

Also by David Drum:

The Chronic Pain Management Sourcebook

Making the Chemotherapy Decision

The Type 2 Diabetes Sourcebook

Second Edition

David Drum and
Terry Zierenberg, R.N., C.D.E.

Foreword by
Calvin Ezrin, M.D.

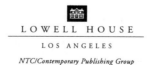

LOWELL HOUSE

LOS ANGELES

NTC/Contemporary Publishing Group

Library of Congress Cataloging-in-Publication Data

Drum, David E.
    The type 2 diabetes sourcebook / by David Drum and Terry Zierenberg.—2nd ed.
      p. cm.
    Includes index.
    ISBN 0-7373-0385-9
     1. Non-insulin-dependent diabetes—Popular works. I. Title: Type two diabetes
sourcebook. II. Zierenberg, Terry. III. Title.

RC662.18 .D78 2000
616.4´62—dc21

00-029894

Published by Lowell House
A division of NTC/Contemporary Publishing Group, Inc.
4255 West Touhy Avenue, Lincolnwood, Illinois 60712, U.S.A.

Printed in the United States of America

International Standard Book Number: 0-7373-0385-9

00 01 02 03 04 DHD 18 17 16 15 14 13 12 11 10 9 8 7 6 5 4 3 2 1

To my grandmother, Mrs. L.A. McInnell

To Robert P. Rood, M.D., whose passion for teaching
has been my inspiration

And in memory of Roxanne Godden, R.N.

CONTENTS

FOREWORD

Successful treatment of Type 2 diabetes carries the promise of delaying the further advance of the tissue damage caused by diabetes and, in some cases, the reversal of it. Good control of diabetes depends so much on a knowledgeable and motivated patient, and *The Type 2 Diabetes Sourcebook* provides a powerful educational tool. There is an increasing worldwide epidemic of Type 2 diabetes, which is usually associated with obesity. Because of its insidious onset, diabetic complications in many cases may be significantly advanced by the time it is diagnosed.

There are now a number of drugs recommended for the treatment of Type 2 diabetes. These supplementary medications work best in a setting of beneficial diet and exercise. If sensible and nonthreatening recommendations for lifestyle changes are applied diligently, there will be less of a need for drugs to control diabetes. *The Type 2 Diabetes Sourcebook* admirably covers the many practical aspects that a person with Type 2 diabetes must address in order to achieve a long and healthy life.

The Type 2 Diabetes Sourcebook represents the collective experience of an outstanding diabetes educator, Terry Zierenberg, and her very capable staff associated with the Diabetes Care Center at the Encino-Tarzana Regional Medical Center, Tarzana, California. Along with David Drum, a skillful medical writer, they have set out important facts duly arranged in simplified language for ready understanding. I foresee this book as a valuable ally for patients and their doctors to combat a major threat to the successful management of this most common and costly form of diabetes—lack of knowledge.

CALVIN EZRIN, M.D.
author of *The Type 2 Diabetes Diet Book* with Robert E. Kowalski

ACKNOWLEDGMENTS

The authors would like to thank the following individuals in the health-care community who provided generous support and useful advice during the preparation of this manuscript: Calvin Ezrin, M.D.; Linda B. Gledhill, Area Executive Director, Western Region, American Diabetes Association, Los Angeles; Helenbeth Reynolds, R.D., University of Minnesota, for the American Dietetic Association; Steve Degelsmith, Ph.D., M.F.C.C., Conflict Solutions and Consultations, Granada Hills, California; Therese Farrell, M.S., R.D., C.D.E., Encino-Tarzana Hospital, Tarzana, California; Josie Curran, R.N., Encino-Tarzana Hospital; Diane Woods, M.S., R.D., C.D.E., Encino-Tarzana Hospital; Debbie Solomin, M.P.H., R.D., Encino-Tarzana Hospital; Terri Hansen, R.N., C.D.E., Glendale Adventist Medical Center, Glendale, California; Roger Curtis, Sitcur Analysis, Los Angeles; Los Angeles insurance brokers Elaine Fried and Howard Fried, The Howard Fried Agency, Alhambra, California; pharmacist Allen Silverman, Tarzana Pharmacy; Jean Partamian, M.D., Richard David, M.D., David Kayne, M.D., Debbie Rehman-Lux, M.F.C.C., Diane Gilman, D.P.M., David Aizuss, M.D., Robert P. Rood, M.D., Yehuda Handelsman, M.D., Julius Griffin, M.D., Norman Lavin, M.D., Paul Sogol, M.D., and the Diabetes Care Center staff at Encino-Tarzana Regional Medical Center, Tarzana, California.

The Type 2 Diabetes Sourcebook

Chapter 1

ABOUT DIABETES

Diabetes Is a Chronic Disease That Can Be Controlled

~

DIABETES IS INVISIBLE, A CHRONIC DISEASE THAT DOES NOT GO AWAY. DIABETES IS NOT like a broken arm—it can't be seen and will never completely heal. Diabetes is a disease that can only be managed. Although you can live a long, full life with diabetes, the disease will affect the way you and your family live. But take comfort in knowing that diabetes is one disease over which you, the patient, can exercise an enormous amount of control.

In this thoroughly revised new edition, the emphasis remains on the control of diabetes through *self-management*, which may be achieved for many years. Self-management means that you choose to participate in your own medical care and in the management of your disease. The first step you take will probably involve simple changes in your lifestyle, rather than exotic medical treatments. If you have just been diagnosed with diabetes, be assured that you have plenty of time to learn how to take good care of yourself, because diabetes progresses very slowly in the body. Diabetes will not kill you today or tomorrow. In fact, although it is a serious disease, diabetes is rarely listed as a cause of death on death certificates.

Even if you have been recently diagnosed with Type 2 diabetes, you have probably been living with it for several years. Frequently, diabetes is not even diagnosed until it is detected by a routine blood test or by the onset of symptoms, such as a slowly healing infection, which can lead a knowledgeable medical doctor or a dentist to suspect the presence of diabetes. Unfortunately, the symptoms of diabetes are so subtle that they can slip past the radar, practically unnoticed, for many years in an otherwise healthy person.

The first thing you can do to help yourself is to visit a medical doctor and be diagnosed with diabetes. This knowledge allows you to take action, to focus on learning more about the disease, and to control its effects. Your primary source of information about the treatment of your diabetes or any other medical condition should be your medical doctor and your medical treatment team. Unfortunately, given the seismic shifts currently underway in our health-care delivery system, your doctor may not have the time to explain the rationale for each aspect of your treatment right away.

In diabetes, treatment typically involves changes in diet, the adoption of a more physically active lifestyle, and sometimes drugs. Stress reduction is an acknowledged component of diabetes care, and one dealt with at length in this book. Unfortunately, many physicians have little time to provide guidance in this area, since stress management is unique to every individual, and is beyond the primary area of expertise of many doctors. Regular visits to medical specialists and a program of daily hygiene are important in your care.

The management of diabetes may seem overwhelmingly complicated at first. It is not.

This book is designed to supplement, not replace, the good advice you receive from your medical team. It will teach you some basic facts about diabetes, a condition that may seem bewildering and foreign to you, especially at first. This book explains which medical treatments and referrals you should expect, including important treatment recommendations established by the American Diabetes Association. It also suggests ways in which you may work as a partner with your doctor and your medical team to apply the best available strategies of diet, exercise, and medication to achieve optimum health.

Diabetes is a time-intensive disease for both doctors and patients. It is widely acknowledged that good diabetes care rests on a foundation of patient knowledge. Unfortunately, some health insurance plans are curtailing rather than increasing their payments to health-care providers for vital educational services. In the current cost-cutting environment, which includes a shift toward managed care, the responsibility for at least a portion of your education about diabetes is frequently handed back to you.

Since Type 2 diabetes appears and is treated differently than Type 1 diabetes, books attempting to cover both types can confuse the reader. Each reader is, after all, dealing with one unique case of diabetes. For this reason, this book deals only with the treatment of Type 2 diabetes. Throughout much of this book, Type 2 diabetes is simply referred to as diabetes. Some medical and scientific terms have been simplified to avoid reader confusion. Every attempt has been made to make this information as accurate and up-to-date as possible.

Fortunately, major advances in the management of diabetes have been made in the past century. Some of the greatest advances have occurred within the past twenty years. After 1980, for instance, advances in technology have allowed patients to monitor the levels of the important blood sugar, glucose, in the privacy of their own homes. Although the first glucose testing devices were large and cumbersome, digital and computer technology, miniaturization, and other improvements have produced an extremely simple, accurate, and lightweight tool that instantly checks the status of the patient's health. Simply knowing the level of glucose in your blood gives you, the patient, the basis to control your disease. Other innovations in diabetes care include new medical treatment techniques and improved medications developed by pharmaceutical companies. Information about diabetes is more available to the average person than ever before.

THE IMPACT OF DIABETES

The American Diabetes Association estimates that one of every five Americans will contract diabetes in their lifetime. In the United States, another person is diagnosed with diabetes every sixty seconds. More than 625,000 new cases of diabetes are diagnosed in the United States each year. An estimated 120 million people in the world—including 16 million Americans—are believed to have diabetes. In the United States, only about half of the estimated cases have actually been diagnosed. It is believed that approximately 8 million people currently suffering from diabetes don't realize that they have the disease. All of these undiagnosed people have Type 2 diabetes.

The financial impact of diabetes is estimated at $92 billion per year by the National Institutes of Health. This estimate includes direct medical costs totaling $45 billion, and indirect costs, such as work loss, disability, and premature death, totaling $47 billion. Diabetes is the sixth most common cause of death by disease in the United States, with an estimated 400,000 deaths per year occurring in people known to have diabetes. Complications that can arise from diabetes make it the leading cause of blindness, kidney disease, amputations, and heart disease. Because of this enormous and growing impact on American health, the United States spends about $12 billion on diabetes research each year, and this research continues to pay off.

Your own diagnosis of diabetes may have unsettled, shocked, or upset you. You will soon move past this period of grieving, which is quite natural and only an expression of your humanity. But first, you must accept that you have a serious disease. You must learn something about diabetes. Then you must manage it intelligently, with as much grace and self-discipline as you can muster each day. It is possible to live a normal, satisfying life with diabetes. Millions of people are accomplishing just that at this very moment.

As later chapters will explain, self-management will take a bit of time and effort each day. Take comfort in knowing that scientific research shows that the time you invest in yourself will improve your health and your quality of life now and in the future. Good self-management cannot only make your life better right now, but it may also slow—or even stop—the progress of complications such as heart disease, which may develop later on.

A diagnosis of diabetes is not a death sentence, but it may be an intimation of your own mortality. It is a fact of life that every living thing is mortal. If you're having trouble dealing with the idea that you have diabetes, try to accept your own mortality, and work backward from there. Look at it this way: With or without diabetes, you may live 80, 90, even 100 years, but you cannot expect to live forever. That you have diabetes is merely a fact of your life. You may learn how to manage the disease in a way that improves the length and the quality of your life. Therefore, it makes a lot of sense to simply accept the fact that you have a disease, and then manage its effects as wisely as you can.

Accepting diabetes is a process. You will surely go through a period of grieving, which may include strong emotions, such as anger, fear, or depression. But those powerful emotions will pass. Understanding diabetes and how to manage it is the next step, one you will make with the help of your doctor and medical team. Good self-management requires education, and then the application of effort, patience, and tenacity. Ultimately, your own continuing efforts will empower you.

WHO GETS DIABETES?

A number of risk factors are known to exist for diabetes. Type 2 diabetes most frequently strikes men and women with a family history of diabetes, people who are over forty years of age, and people who are overweight. Women who have a baby that weighs more than nine pounds are frequently at risk for developing Type 2 diabetes, even if the diabetes that developed during pregnancy goes away after the baby is born. Sedentary lifestyles, physical stress, emotional stress, and high-fat diets are recognized risk factors. A medical condition called impaired glucose tolerance, present in 11 percent of adults, is another identified risk factor for Type 2 diabetes.

Although people from all ethnic groups are diagnosed with diabetes, Latinos, African Americans, Asian Americans, and Native Americans are statistically much more likely to have it. In some American Indian communities, more than half of the adults have Type 2 diabetes; pregnant women in those communities have an extraordinarily high incidence of gestational diabetes of 14 percent. The average person diagnosed with Type 2 diabetes is between fifty-five and sixty years old. Although uncommon, people under the age of twenty-five are also diagnosed with Type 2 diabetes, which is one reason that the disease is no longer called maturity onset diabetes, the more descriptive name it bore for years.

Diabetes is a disease that may be rooted in industrial progress. Even today, it is rare in so-called developing countries. However, statistical studies show that as countries develop an industrial base, the incidence of diabetes skyrockets. This upsurge in the incidence of diabetes occurred first in Japan after World War II, and has more recently appeared in Korea, Taiwan, and other industrializing Asian countries. That greater numbers of people in these countries suddenly began to be diagnosed with diabetes indicates that something associated with industrialization brought their latent diabetes into full bloom. Industrial progress is often accompanied by massive shifts in eating patterns; whole populations stop eating simple foods such as black bread, rice, and tortillas and begin consuming larger quantities of more complex food products, such as meat and milk from domesticated animals, and more processed and conveniently packaged food products. In addition, the most privileged citizens of newly affluent lands quickly assume the sedentary, exercise-free lifestyle that passes for luxury in our time—a lifestyle that may help set them up for a diagnosis of diabetes.

Medical doctors have been able to diagnose diabetes for centuries. However, most of the advances in the treatment of diabetes have occurred in the twentieth century. Insulin, for instance, was not discovered until 1921. Many advances in diabetes care have come about because of the sophistication of our measuring devices, which allow medical doctors to measure small quantities of chemicals such as glucose, cholesterol, and damaged proteins in the blood. It was only in 1979 that the National Diabetes Data Group concluded that there were actually two basic classifications for diabetes—Type 1, in which absolutely no insulin is produced in the body, and Type 2, in which insulin is produced but not properly utilized by the body.

WHO GETS DIABETES?

According to the American Diabetes Association, the chances of having diabetes are as follows:

GROUP	AGE	INCIDENCE
All people	lifetime	1 in 5
Anglos	20–44	1 in 62
Anglos	45–74	1 in 8
African Americans	25–44	1 in 25
African Americans	45–54	1 in 14
African Americans	55–64	1 in 4
African Americans	65–74	1 in 7
Latinos	20–44	1 in 16
Latinos	45–74	1 in 3.5

ABOUT THIS BOOK

It helps to think of yourself not as a victim of diabetes but as a person with diabetes who has choices to make. As you will see, making good choices may literally change your life.

This newly revised book may help empower you by providing you with useful information in several crucial areas. While it is *not* intended to replace the medical advice of the doctor who treats your diabetes, or the recommendations of other specialists whom you consult, this book will explain ways in which you might consider changing your lifestyle to help manage the effects of diabetes. On a very human level, this book includes case histories of people who are now living with diabetes. This book provides useful suggestions for coping with the physical and mental ramifications of the disease.

This chapter provides an introduction to diabetes, an overview of the book, and an explanation of who is most likely to contract the disease.

Chapter 2 discusses empowerment, explaining how men and women with diabetes may choose to take some control over the management of this disease.

Chapter 3 discusses your interactions with the medical system, including tips on building a partnership with your doctor, and selecting a good health-care team. Chapter 3 also contains the American Diabetes Association's "Bill of Rights," which recommends specific standards of treatment you should expect from your doctor.

Chapter 4 explains the basic biology of Type 2 diabetes.

Chapter 5 discusses the vitally important principle of self-management, the most important concept of all because the day-to-day management of diabetes is up to you. Chapter 5 also contains techniques and methods for dealing with the greater levels of physical and emotional stress that you may encounter when living with this disease.

Chapter 6 discusses your single most important self-management tool, blood glucose testing. This chapter takes you through a step-by-step explanation of the simple equipment you may purchase and use to track your blood glucose levels, and suggests ways to use testing to achieve better health.

Chapter 7, the longest chapter in the book, addresses the important area of nutrition, an aspect of self-management that is important for all people. This chapter also contains a number of strategies and tips for changing your eating style.

Chapter 8 focuses on developing a more physically active lifestyle, another change that has been proven to help control blood sugar. Strategies for incorporating more physical activity and exercise into your life are discussed, as are some simple precautions to be taken with any program of exercise.

Chapter 9 deals with the drugs prescribed by doctors to help patients manage their diabetes, including the newest diabetes drugs, such as metformin, pioglitazone, and acarbose as well as more established medications such as insulin.

Chapter 10 looks at the standard laboratory tests you may take at your doctor's office, and explains what the results may mean to you.

Chapter 11 discusses the day-to-day management of diabetes, including many of the simple steps of hygiene and preventive maintenance that you can take to prevent medical problems before they occur. This chapter also discusses how to care for yourself on sick days.

Chapter 12 looks at diabetes that develops during pregnancy, and includes some tips for keeping yourself healthy.

Chapter 13 discusses the often-neglected emotional and social effects of diabetes, which involve you, your family, and friends. This chapter includes suggestions for improving communication between you and your family and friends, and guidelines for working with a mental health professional or a diabetes support group.

Chapter 14 discusses the financial aspects of diabetes, including an estimate of the costs you may incur. Also included are tips on working with health insurance companies and Medicare, and suggestions for buying supplies.

Chapter 15 looks at the long-term complications of diabetes, including information on the latest strategies for treatment.

Chapter 16 deals with self-management over the long run, and examines some promising developments in diabetes research.

Additional information is included in two appendixes at the back of the book. Appendix A lists some of the resources available for people with diabetes, including addresses and toll-free telephone numbers for educational, professional, and volunteer organizations. The second appendix, a glossary of diabetes terms, is intended to help demystify some of the medical jargon you may encounter.

GOOD HEALTH

Achieving good health involves more than merely treating a particular disease. For this reason, the best medical treatment these days utilizes a multidisciplinary approach, which focuses treatment on the whole person rather than on the physical body alone. This "whole person" approach is the philosophy behind this book.

Although the topic of this book is Type 2 diabetes, ultimately this book aims to teach you how to maintain and maximize your good health in the fullest sense of the word. Good health, after all, isn't just something you think about when you get diabetes. Good health involves the entire person, and includes both physical and mental health.

Remember that the World Health Organization has defined health as "the complete state of physical, mental, and social well-being, not merely the absence of disease."

With this definition in mind, we turn first to the cornerstone of good diabetes care—empowerment. In the next chapter, learn how the empowering spotlight of good self-management can shine its bright, healing beam upon you.

Chapter 2

EMPOWERMENT

How You Can Help Yourself

~

MANY PEOPLE LIVE QUITE SUCCESSFULLY WITH DIABETES. ONE ASPECT OF THIS IS empowerment. Empowerment involves your choice to take a measure of control over your own life. This chapter introduces the concept of empowerment, an attitude that can embrace every aspect of your diabetes treatment. Empowerment may involve working with your health-care team, and working with family and friends. But most of all, empowerment involves a continuing process of educating yourself, and working with you.

Don't think for one moment that a diagnosis of diabetes means that you can't live a rich, full, productive, fun-loving, even quite extraordinary life. Tennis star Billy Talbert, baseball champions Jackie Robinson and Catfish Hunter, and hockey star Bobby Clarke didn't let the fact that they had diabetes stop them from excelling in brutally competitive professional sports. Diabetes did not compromise the brilliant show business careers of comedians Jack Benny and Mary Tyler Moore or vocalist Ella Fitzgerald. Businessman Ray Kroc didn't let diabetes stop him from parlaying one little hamburger stand into the world's largest and most successful fast-food chain—McDonald's. Although U.S. Supreme Court Chief Justice Oliver Wendell Holmes had diabetes, he wrote many brilliant and well-researched legal opinions before he died at the age of ninety-four.

It is possible to see diabetes as a challenge, one that may become a turning point in your life. Weight lifter Ron Gillembardo began lifting weights after he was diagnosed with Type 2 diabetes at the age of thirty-eight. This inspired him to lose 100 pounds in two years. Gillembardo's exercise of choice, weight lifting, sparked a continuing passion that led him, at the age of forty-five, to become the oldest man in history ever to compete in the powerlifting event in the 1992 Barcelona Olympics—an accomplishment he now attributes to his diagnosis of diabetes.

The old joke about psychologists also relates directly to the concept of empowerment.

Question: "How many psychologists does it take to change a light bulb?"

Answer: "Only one, but the light bulb has got to want to be changed."

Empowerment means learning about and managing at least some aspects of your diabetes. Unfortunately, some people believe that health care is solely their doctors' responsibility. The problem with this attitude is that diabetes cannot be cured with a prescription for medicine, an elaborate machine, or even a surgical operation. Diabetes is not a death sentence, but it is a long-haul, long-term disease. Living with diabetes is a lot more like running a marathon than running a 100-yard dash.

The good news is that you begin to empower yourself the moment you begin to participate in your own health care. Your own efforts may make a huge difference both day-to-day and over the long term.

The best news about diabetes is that you can make a big impact on the course of the disease. To make a difference, you will need to practice good *self-management*. You have a choice about whether or not you wish to become involved in your own health. Although it may not be simple or easy, self-management can be integrated into your life, and even become routine, as the following story illustrates.

RUTH'S STORY

Twelve years ago, when she reached the age of thirty-eight, a woman we shall call Ruth was diagnosed with Type 2 diabetes. The news frightened and shocked this mother of two children. She was in the midst of a bustling, busy, productive life.

"I was scared," Ruth remembers. "I asked, 'Why me?' I wondered if it was a death sentence for me."

In retrospect, Ruth suspected something was amiss. When she was sixteen, a doctor told her she had "a touch of sugar" in her blood, gave her diabetes pills for a year and a half, then pronounced her "cured." At twenty, a physician mentioned in passing that she was "borderline diabetic." When she was pregnant at twenty-four, another doctor told her she was "slightly diabetic," but reassured her the diabetes would go away after her pregnancy.

But the blood tests confirmed that Ruth had Type 2 diabetes, a disease that ran in her family—a disease she knew little about.

At her doctor's suggestion, Ruth attended educational classes in which the importance of blood sugar testing, nutrition, and diet were explained, as were the possible complications of diabetes.

"I was scared when I went in, and the educational classes were even scarier," Ruth remembers. "They talked about the neuropathy, the blindness, and other complications. I thought it was all going to happen right then and there. About that time, my gynecologist learned that I had diabetes; he said I would have to remove my

IUD, and suggested I get my tubes tied. All of a sudden I felt like this high-risk person. It was overwhelming."

Then Ruth's mother, who had never talked much about her own diabetes, died. Ruth's life "got all mixed up," and she endured great emotional stress.

Ruth got wind of a diabetes support group that met in a nearby town. One evening, she attended a meeting. Although she was frightened, she liked the people in the group, and was encouraged to come back. Over the years, the group has become an important part of Ruth's personal support system. When she began attending support group meetings, she was taking diabetes pills and working to change her diet, but was afraid to begin glucose testing at home.

"At the time, I was afraid to stick my finger," Ruth recalls. "One thing that the support group helped with was explaining to me that the finger would only hurt for a second, but that I could hurt myself for life by not pricking my finger. I had a hard time with this at first. I used to meditate before pricking my finger. It took a few years before I came to a total acceptance of it."

Another part of Ruth's support system has been a knowledgeable and supportive physician. The doctor who treats her is an endocrinologist and doctor of internal medicine who specializes in the care of diabetes. She says his caring attitude reminds her of an old-time family doctor who made house calls. Ruth has learned how important it is to be honest with her doctor, particularly about the results of blood sugar tests.

She admits it took her some time to adjust to the ups and downs of blood sugar testing results.

"I used to wonder why I couldn't get the numbers right," she recalls. "I used to feel so frustrated that I was doing things right, but the numbers would come out wrong. For instance, I'd eat the same thing one day as I did the day before, and the numbers would come out different. Finally, I realized it's not a right or wrong kind of thing. I know now that you can do everything right and things can still go haywire. It's a constant roller coaster ride, and constantly changing."

As she became more accomplished at self-management, Ruth swept like a tornado through her personal life, a super mom who worked full-time as an accountant, held a second job, raised two children as a single parent, attended college classes, sat on a hospital board, and maintained an active dating life.

But five years after being diagnosed with diabetes, about the time her doctor wanted her to begin taking insulin, Ruth suffered a major heart attack. This knocked her down into a depression.

"To be stopped in my tracks with a heart attack was devastating ...to be forty-three years old and to have a major heart attack. I felt I couldn't do anything," she recalls.

A mental health professional helped her move through this crisis in her life.

During Ruth's recovery from the heart attack, she received help and encouragement from her diabetes support group. She was having to kick her newspaper from her front porch into the house with her feet, since she was not allowed to bend over to pick it up. A friend from the support group brought her a "grabber" device to help her pick up the newspaper, and to help her reach other things around the house. Her doctor started her on a newly approved diabetes medication, Glucophage, which allowed her to lower the amount of insulin she took each day.

Ruth asked for help from her support group when she began insulin, and she got it. Taking insulin has now become as routine for her as blood testing.

"I sure wish I didn't have diabetes, but it's become a part of my life," Ruth says. "I have finally reached a point where I feel like my life has some form of balance. I reached a point where I could accept it. Now I take insulin and test my blood sugar just like I go to the bathroom and brush my teeth. Today, it would almost be strange *not* to do those things. By learning how to take care of situations like high or low blood sugar, I get a sense of being safe and secure. The more I know, the better off I am. It's very important to keep learning and to keep growing."

RESPONSIBILITY

Diabetes puts responsibility on you. This responsibility may be frightening at first, particularly if you're still grappling with the idea of having a chronic disease. Fortunately, the progress of diabetes is slow. If you choose to educate yourself, you have adequate time to learn. When you understand how to manage and control the effects of diabetes, your knowledge will empower you, and perhaps your family. Good self-management of diabetes may actually become routine.

Whenever you choose to do so, you can educate yourself. You can assess where you are, what you have gone through, and what may lie ahead.

With the help of medical professionals, you can take control of the day-to-day management of your disease. Your participation helps your health-care team develop a treatment plan that is appropriate to you, and your life as you live it right now. You can work at your own pace to adopt a healthy, affirming lifestyle that may greatly improve the quality of your life.

Although Western culture worships individualism, when it comes to diabetes, it's not always best to try to tough it out alone. In fact, most people do a better job of maintaining their overall health (and dealing with diabetes) if they have emotional support from friends, family, or a diabetes support group. Recent research conducted at the University of Hawaii by Chen-Yen Wang and Mildred Fenske has verified the important role of social support in overall health. Within a group of men and women with Type 2 diabetes, those who had a supportive family member, a diabetes support group, or even a sympathetic friend did significantly better both in caring for their own overall health and in managing their diabetes. As shown on page 20, those who took the best care of themselves had both a supportive family and a diabetes support group. People with no social or emotional support took the poorest care of themselves. The moral of this research is that it may actually benefit your health if you communicate what you're doing with a sympathetic family member or friend, or find a good diabetes support group to help you along your way.

A BELIEF SYSTEM

A therapist experienced in working with people who have diabetes defines empowerment as "a belief system that involves having the tools, and feeling competent and effective in what you're doing and how you do it." The emotional and physical benefits that accompany empowerment are immense.

Certainly, thinking of yourself as a victim without any choices to make in your life doesn't work. Yes, you have diabetes, probably because you had a genetic predisposition to the disease. Diabetes is merely a fact of your life, not your life itself. No matter what the future holds, you will continue to have choices to make in your own life, including fundamental choices about how much you wish to participate in your own care. Simply educating yourself about diabetes and then practicing good self-management can improve your health, save you money, and yield a higher-quality life.

Some of the benefits of good self-management may cause better health in the future. The recent United Kingdom Prospective Diabetes Study, or UKPDS, a large twenty-year trial completed in 1997, involved more than 5,000 Britons who began the trial newly diagnosed with Type 2 diabetes. It showed that the members of the group that maintained tight glucose control—that is, kept their blood sugar levels as near as possible to normal—significantly reduced their risk of complications. In one part of the trial, two groups were asked to follow a low-fat, high-fiber diet, with half of all calories ingested in carbohydrate form. One group was also treated with diabetes drugs or insulin, and given instructions on how to achieve good control. Compared to the group receiving only dietary treatment, the group members with tight control achieved an 11 percent reduction in important HbA1c test levels. They achieved a 25 percent reduction in risk of small blood vessel complications, especially eye problems. They also reduced their risk of heart attacks by 16 percent.

BENEFITS OF SOCIAL SUPPORT

Social support makes people more likely to participate in their own health care, according to a recent study of the influence of family and friends on a group of people with Type 2 diabetes.

The difference between mean compliance scores among people with various types of social support and those without support is listed below:

Compliance in General Health Care

Type of Support	vs. No Support
Support of family plus friend	22% higher
Support of family plus support group	17% higher
Support of family	17% higher
Support of friend plus support group	8% higher
Support of friend	4% higher

Compliance in Diabetes Self-Management

Type of Support	vs. No Support
Support of family plus support group	35% higher
Support of family plus friend	27% higher
Support of family	22% higher
Support of friend plus support group	10% higher
Support of friend only	1% higher

Source: The Diabetes Educator, September/October 1996.

In another part of the trial, people with Type 2 diabetes who had high blood pressure were instructed to check their blood pressure regularly and to use drugs to reduce blood pressure. After nine years, the group whose blood pressure was more tightly controlled had a significantly lower incidence of complications including heart attack, stroke, and eye problems. This 24 percent reduction in diabetes-related complications and 37 percent reduction in small blood vessel complications led the authors to state "the management of blood pressure should have a high priority in the treatment of Type 2 diabetes."

Robert Turner, M.D., who headed the British study, said, "We know now that if we aim for lower-to-normal blood glucose concentration, and near-to-normal blood pressure, then it is possible to reduce the risk of complications and maintain the health of the patient. It's not that we need a new treatment. We can use the present treatments that are available more intensively."

In the United States, the seven-year Diabetes Control and Complications Trial, completed in 1993, led to similar conclusions about the importance of good blood sugar control of a large group of people with Type 1 diabetes. This trial showed a 60 percent reduction in incidents of eye disease, kidney disease, and nerve damage and a delayed onset of complications when blood sugar was tightly controlled.

Good results were achieved in all subjects, regardless of age, gender, or duration of diabetes.

While it is not certain that these results apply across the board to people with Type 2 diabetes, the American Diabetes Association is convinced enough to recommend strict control for most people with Type 2 diabetes. A similar research trial involving people with Type 2 diabetes is underway in research centers across the United States.

A FORK IN THE ROAD

At this moment, think of yourself at a crossroads in your life. Visualize yourself as a little boy or girl carrying a bag of groceries home from the store. You come to a fork in the road. To the left is a rather shadowy road marked by a sign reading Poor Self-Management. Down the crooked, winding road of Poor Self-Management lives a gang of unruly kids called the Complications—Heart Disease, Blindness, Amputations, Kidney Problems, and Neuropathy. To the right is another fork in the road, better illuminated with a sign reading Good Self-Management. The Complications gang only occasionally ventures onto the road to Good Self-Management because the bright lights usually keep it away. You may be at a fork in that road right now. It's your choice as to which way you will turn.

Successful self-management involves a measure of listening to your own body. You'll need to develop an ability to listen to the messages your body sends to you, indirectly in the form of feelings and symptoms that may be subtle, and directly in the form of blood sugar readings and test results. As a general rule, the more you and your health-care team can tailor your self-management to fit your life, the more successful your self-management of diabetes—and your own empowerment—will be.

OVERCOMING OBSTACLES

Take a moment to reflect on the events of your life. If you've lived a few decades, you have already overcome some obstacles and setbacks. You have won victories. You have gathered the strength you needed at important times. As you empower yourself through the concept of self-management, take a moment to recall your personal victories, and recount some of the things you have already accomplished, already achieved, or already won.

Diabetes is simply one area of your life in which you can choose to help yourself. Yes, it may well take an expenditure of will. Perhaps it will require a continuing display of personal courage. Self-management involves you, your doctors, your medical team, your social circle, and the greater world. Self-management involves learning a little bit of science, and applying this knowledge adroitly to yourself. Yes, this process will take education, time, and energy. It may require self-discipline, manual dexterity, and some emotional strength. Diabetes will affect the way you live your life. But you can make the necessary changes.

It is even possible that you may become a better and stronger person, because your efforts may become one of the turning points of your life.

BEYOND GRIEVING

Accepting that you have diabetes, and that you are not quite as healthy as you thought you were, involves a process of grieving. It is normal to ache with grief when you experience or anticipate the loss of something precious to you. Many persons diagnosed with a chronic disease experience a profound grief, an intimation of their own mortality that is better seen as an emotional process than a single, isolated event. According to author and research psychiatrist Elisabeth Kübler-Ross, who has long studied the emotional aspects of serious illness, the process of grieving often involves a series of emotional changes or plateaus. The attendant emotional turmoil may include an initial shock or denial, followed by anger, guilt or bargaining, depression, and eventually acceptance. But hope is a constant in this process because it allows us to look past the present moment toward something better. The way each person handles and moves through grieving varies, but weathering this emotional process can be the first step to accepting and then to managing your disease.

With diabetes, you may worry about your health on a practical, everyday level—fretting that you aren't getting the details right, that you're not being "a good diabetic" every day in every way. You may become upset when you discover a gap in your knowledge that takes time or effort to fill. Or you may simply have to allow yourself some time to adjust to the big changes that have muscled their way into your life. Accept that some aspects of self-management may be emotionally

STEPS TO EMPOWER YOURSELF

Here are a few general ways in which you can empower yourself:

- Identify your own attitudes about learning more about the management of diabetes, particularly your own feelings about accepting a measure of responsibility for it. If you resent having diabetes, for instance, admit that you resent it and then move on.
- Learn more about Type 2 diabetes, including how you and your health-care team can better manage its effects.
- Put something you have learned into practice today.
- Periodically record your efforts in a record book or on a chart.
- Share your successes with other people who have diabetes—family members, friends, or members of a support group. Keeping a written diary or seeing a therapist may be helpful in some cases.
- Realize that your life has other aspects such as work, children, or family which are more important to you than the management of your diabetes.

or physically stressful, particularly at first, during the most emotionally vulnerable times.

Putting attitudes about diabetes to rest among family or friends is not always a picnic, either, particularly if they seem to be overly worried about you or simply don't seem to share your level of concern. Something as simple as beginning an exercise program or changing the recipe for a dish served at holiday meals may spark heated family arguments and stir up emotional stress. These aspects of diabetes may seem quite overwhelming. Diabetes may add greater stress to your life.

The best news is that you can learn to manage negative stress. This is quite important because stress directly affects your body in a harmful way—by jacking up your blood sugar. Relieving stress can benefit your health almost immediately by helping to bring your blood sugar levels down. As explained in chapter 5, you may learn ways to relieve the stress associated with diabetes, one aspect of giving yourself a more pleasant and more manageable life.

At first, the medical issues may seem very complex. Rest assured that you can understand everything you really need to know if you begin to educate yourself, and then make an effort to continue learning. Working with your doctor and a good diabetes educator will help you understand how your body works, what symptoms you must watch for, and how to handle the various questions and problems that arise. Before you know it, you may well become the family expert on diabetes.

A PROCESS OF MASTERY

Another way to define empowerment is "a process by which people gain mastery over their affairs." In the case of diabetes, this empowering process involves self-management, discussed at greater length beginning in chapter 5. At its best, the self-management process will energize and inspire you because you will gain a measure of control over your own destiny. This will help and empower you.

Medical treatment is somewhat more difficult to accept with a chronic disease than it is with a simple medical problem such as a case of strep throat. You take the antibiotics your doctor prescribes to clear up the strep throat, and your payoff is immediate. Your sore throat feels better because the infection has healed. With diabetes, the reward for taking good care of yourself is that you only feel about the same. The physical "payoff" isn't as immediate or as visible as the disappearance of a sore throat. In an age of instant gratification, diabetes is one of the great frustrations. Self-management is something you must patiently work into the fabric of your life without a lot of payback. You must accept, through a combination of knowledge and faith, that your efforts are worthwhile because self-management lacks immediate, tangible rewards.

In the beginning especially, accepting some responsibility for your health can be frustrating, fraught with emotion, and hampered by the grieving process that is normal after any bad medical news. True, you will never have to live like Nathaniel Hawthorne's Puritan-era heroine, Hester Prynne, by wearing a big red D around your neck that marks you as a person with diabetes. For the moment, accept the idea that empowerment might liberate you because it gives you the knowledge to help yourself.

EDUCATING YOURSELF

When they choose to participate in the process, many people succeed in following many or all of the recommendations given to them by health-care professionals. This educational give-and-take is best seen as a partnership between you and your health-care team, not like the trips the ancient Greeks made to the Oracle of Delphi, where they knelt in the darkness to receive words of wisdom and prophecy from the gods. Keeping yourself healthy is a time-consuming process, and it can be frustrating, but it is also an educational process that should continue for your entire life.

Excellent diabetes educational programs exist all over the world, offering group or individual instruction. The U.S. Center for Disease Control in Atlanta estimates that for every dollar spent on outpatient education, between two and three dollars are saved in hospitalization costs alone. Some of the best diabetes educational programs are for inpatients in the hospital; other good programs, designed for outpatients, are open to the public for a reasonable fee. Most major diabetes centers in the United States offer these programs, as do many clinics, hospitals, and some health maintenance organizations. To continue learning, you may also join the local affiliate of the American Diabetes

Association. This can be quite useful, since most affiliates have periodic educational meetings, workshops, or panel discussions that feature guest speakers and experts who can answer your questions. The American Diabetes Association is always looking for volunteers. Support groups for people with diabetes are another way to educate and empower yourself.

Outside of these formal settings, you can read books, go to the library, subscribe to magazines specializing in diabetes, or even take it upon yourself to search the burgeoning informational databases and newsgroups on the Internet and the World Wide Web.

Empowerment is both an art and a science. The science involves such necessary skills as checking your own glucose levels and understanding your test results. The art involves integrating what you learn as gracefully as possible into your life. You take the first measure of control over your destiny when you choose to help and empower yourself.

Empowerment is an important concept that begins with your education and ultimately involves a choice to help yourself. Some support from family and friends will likely help you maintain a good program of self-management. One of the most important factors in developing a program of good self-management is your doctor. Ideally in partnership with you, your doctor leads the group of people who comprise your medical team, the subject of the next chapter.

Chapter 3

TREATMENT

You, Your Health-Care Team, and
the Patient's Bill of Rights

~

THESE DAYS, THE BEST DIABETES CARE INVOLVES A MULTIDISCIPLINARY APPROACH. Specialists from several disciplines deal with the whole person who is you. This chapter includes a brief explanation of some of the people you might find on your medical team, their roles, and what you might expect from them. Tips for selecting a good doctor and a good health-care team are included. Also included is an important checklist of the things that the doctor who treats your diabetes should do on your first visit—the American Diabetes Association's treatment recommendations, known as the Patient's Bill of Rights.

Ideally, a team of specialists will be ready and willing to help you learn the fundamentals of self-management. Headed by your medical doctor, in partnership with you, this team should include a physician who specializes in the care of diabetes—either an internist with advanced training in diabetes, called a *diabetologist,* or a specialist in the endocrine system, called an *endocrinologist.*

Another member of your health-care team may educate you in the day-to-day self-management of diabetes, including the basics of blood glucose testing. This person may be called a *certified diabetes educator, nurse educator,* or *physician-trained assistant.* A *nutritionist* or *registered dietitian* may help you modify your eating style by planning nutritious meals or developing a plan to help you lose weight if that is recommended. Some doctors or diabetes programs also enlist the expertise of an *exercise physiologist,* a specialist in the effects of exercise on the body, who will help you develop a program of physical activity tailored to your abilities and needs. Nurses, dietitians, and exercise specialists may also be certified diabetes educators, which means that they have certified in-depth knowledge of diabetes in addition to their professional training. *Mental health professionals* such as a psychiatrist, psychologist, or social worker may join your team if you have trouble handling the emotional turmoil that sometimes accompanies diabetes.

Rather than maintaining all of these specialists on staff, some doctors refer their patients to good, established diabetes educational programs. Offered through hospitals or clinics, these programs provide classes in basic coping skills, and sometimes host diabetes support groups and ongoing educational programs. Other doctors prefer to handle most of the recommendations for lifestyle changes alone.

Research has shown that a team approach usually works best because each specialist handles an important aspect of your treatment. However it is composed, your medical team should work with you to help empower you and give you the confidence you need to take a hand in your own care.

Any successful program of lifestyle changes, of course, should be built around your needs and involve your participation from the beginning. If you are willing to participate even a little, the treatment plan should incorporate that amount of participation. Some involvement is preferable to none. Your medical team should give you the sense that what you do makes a difference, because it does. A feeling of "buying in" to a partnership with your health-care team should develop quickly. Your desire to follow through with the program that you helped design will be important in the long run.

SELECTING A DOCTOR

You choose your doctor, if not your entire health-care team. If you're enrolled in a health maintenance organization, or HMO, your choice of a doctor to treat your diabetes may be limited, although you probably will have some choice even within the HMO. Most doctors are caring and competent. However, if you absolutely don't like a particular doctor, you can always find a way to visit another doctor. Note that changing doctors will *not* cure diabetes, although it may improve how you feel about your treatment.

Some questions you might want to ask any doctor who treats diabetes include:

- How much specialized medical training have you received in the treatment of diabetes?
- Are you now treating many patients with diabetes?
- How much input do you expect from me during my treatment?
- What is your treatment philosophy regarding lifestyle changes and the use of prescription medications?

Ideally, the doctor who treats your diabetes will have received special training in treating diabetes and will be experienced in treating people who have it. The treatment of Type 2 diabetes involves lifestyle changes and medicines, but lifestyle changes are almost always the preferred first approach. You might want to think twice about a doctor who relies only on medical interventions, such as pills and insulin, and never even considers a holistic approach to diabetes. The best treatment always involves the whole person.

While it's true that some doctors seem to think that M.D. stands for Medical Deity, many physicians are in fact sympathetic people, confident in their ability to help you but also aware of their limitations. Given adequate time and accurate information, a good doctor should be able to clearly analyze the state of your health and give you the tools you need to help yourself, including referrals or suggestions for dietary and lifestyle changes, and medications when necessary. More and more, the ideal relationship between a patient and a physician is being seen as a collaboration, more like a business partnership than the relationship between a vassal and a king.

After you have been diagnosed with diabetes, your doctor will recommend a treatment plan, explaining the risks and benefits of the recommendations. Your doctor only *recommends* a plan to treat your diabetes. You must choose to accept the recommendations. Participating in the creation of your treatment plan will help you integrate it into your life.

Remember that you are a consumer of health-care services, and you should expect to get everything you pay for. Utilizing the combined educational skills of all the people on your medical team broadens the scope of your treatment and can make it more effective. Look for a team that pays attention to you, that treats you like a person and not just another number. The ability of your medical team to tailor your treatment plan to you is a leading indicator of that plan's success.

The Joslin Diabetes Center in Boston, one of the oldest and best in the United States, has prepared the following checklist to help guide people in the selection of a health-care team. This checklist is excerpted from the most recent edition of *The Joslin Guide to Diabetes.*

A GOOD HEALTH-CARE TEAM

- They are knowledgeable about diabetes and its care.
- They listen to your concerns and help you identify solutions to the problems.
- They are sensitive to the challenges of life with diabetes.
- They return phone calls within an appropriate time.
- They consult you and consider your lifestyle, likes, dislikes, and abilities when developing your diabetes-care program.
- They work with you to help maintain the best diabetes control possible.
- They help you learn as much as possible about diabetes and how to prevent complications.
- They routinely perform necessary tests and evaluations.
- In accordance with the findings of the Diabetes Control and Complications Trial, they believe it is very important to keep your blood sugar as close to normal as possible.
- They participate in activities of the American Diabetes Association.

All Joslin Diabetes Centers and their affiliates meet these guidelines, as do other good diabetes programs, medical clinics, and health maintenance organizations in the United States.

When you find a doctor's office or clinic in which you feel comfortable, you may well sense it before you leave the office. Give these professionals a chance to know you, and give yourself a chance to know them. Your confidence in your medical team is an important element in designing a program that you can live with for some time. Your program should eventually come to fit your lifestyle like a comfortable pair of shoes because you will need to practice good self-management for a long time.

Take immediate steps to follow the plan you helped create and communicate any problems you have to your medical team (if a team approach is used in your treatment). Your responsibility includes letting the appropriate person know about any problems you have following the team's recommendations, and asking for suggestions.

The doctor who treats your diabetes will probably spend a lot of time with you on your first visit. After that, come back for follow-up visits as you are asked to do, or for emergencies. Of course, report all medical emergencies at once. Set and keep return appointments with other members of your health-care team. When you don't understand something, assert yourself and get answers you can understand. With their permission, you may tape-record your visits with medical professionals because this may help you to remember the details of what was said.

GOOD LISTENING

Doctors are taught in medical school to listen to what their patients say, but some tend to forget this under the pressures of their work—which involves seeing a great number of patients over the course of a day. The doctor treating your diabetes should *listen* to you, especially on the first visit, because a person who's been living with a disease for years may be expected to have more insight into it than anyone else.

Within reasonable limits, your doctor should be able to answer a few questions during each visit. It's your job to ask the questions and get them answered. For instance, if your doctor says your glycosylated hemoglobin test is "okay" or "a bit high, but acceptable," you might ask for the test results and write them down, or even request a photocopy of the test results. If you're curious, ask your doctor what an ideal result on this test might be for you. You may have to ask for certain information because most doctors have some patients who don't wish to know any of the details of their medical treatment, or who get angry or confused when presented with information they don't understand.

As soon as possible, let your doctor know that you want to be educated about your treatment as much as possible. Many doctors will respond positively to this approach.

Since you may not remember medical information for long, it's a good idea to start your own personal *medical file* containing information about your treatment. Your medical file can contain the date and times you saw particular doctors or specialists, their instructions or recommendations to you, test results, and other pertinent data. Some people chart or graph their test results. Keeping good records gives some individuals a feeling of comfort, since it's easy to feel that your life has spun out of control in a brisk, somewhat impersonal medical system. Printed materials, tape recordings, written instructions from your medical team, drug prescriptions, and other medical information may be kept in this file. The advantage of keeping such a file is that you can easily retrieve the information you've collected because it's all in one place.

Remember, you do not have to adore your doctor, but you should trust his or her ability to treat diabetes. Doctors are human; the best ones will listen and talk honestly to you. However, some aspects of your medical condition may not have clear or easily understood answers, and they may take more time to explain than the doctor has available. But, if you ever lose faith in your doctor's ability to treat you, you have the option of consulting another doctor.

YOUR FIRST VISIT

On your first visit to the doctor who will treat your diabetes, you'll be asked to give or complete a *medical history* of yourself. The medical history should include questions about relatives who might have had diabetes, any symptoms of complications, and medical treatments you've had in the past. Be as honest as possible in answering these questions, even those you find somewhat embarrassing to answer frankly. Accurate information will help your doctor understand your problems and treat you. After your doctor has examined your medical history, you should receive a complete physical examination and certain laboratory tests.

Since the treatment of diabetes is time intensive, your first visit will probably be your longest one with the doctor. Expect to spend some time in the office. If you are anxious about your health, or if you want a little comfort or support, take your spouse, a family member, or a friend along. This person can be your personal advocate. With permission from your doctor, you can let your personal advocate sit in on your visits, since two heads are better than one when it comes to remembering information. You may also tape-record any conversation with your doctor, although you should ask permission in advance. Most doctors have no problem with tape-recording, since they know it helps their patients to remember.

Although you may leave the doctor's office with a lot of information, including brochures and written materials, don't expect to learn everything you will need to know on your first visit. You should be able to schedule follow-up visits to members of your health-care team as needed. If you have questions early on, certified diabetes educators are often a good place to start.

THE PATIENT'S BILL OF RIGHTS

On your first visit, you'll be given a complete physical examination. This examination should follow treatment recommendations set by the American Diabetes Association—sometimes called the Patient's Bill of Rights. A leading professional and volunteer organization based in

Alexandria, Virginia, the American Diabetes Association has a membership that includes medical professionals and volunteers as well as expert physician committees that recommend and set standards for good diabetes care.

According to the Patient's Bill of Rights, a complete medical examination begins with standard measurements of your height, weight, blood pressure, and pulse. You should be asked about your diagnosis of diabetes, related test results, and any complications you've had. In conjunction with this visit, you should be given blood tests and urine tests to check your blood glucose level, your glycosylated hemoglobin level, your cholesterol and fat levels, and the level of protein in your urine. Depending on your age and symptoms, you may also be given other medical tests at this time. For instance, a test of the feet, using a plastic bristle called a monofilament, should be given every one to three years to locate any developing nerve problems early. Robert P. Rood, M.D., notes that the rate of amputations in the United States could be cut in half if every doctor included this test along with an examination of the feet with every physical exam of every person with diabetes. However, he notes that only about 8 percent of doctors actually take the shoes off their patients—a percentage that should be much higher.

The American Diabetes Association recommends that the doctor who treats your diabetes examine your eyes, mouth, hands, fingers, and feet, checking for sensation and pulses. Your doctor should check your skin, especially the places where you may have injected insulin. Your doctor should feel your neck to check your thyroid gland, feel your abdomen to check your liver and other organs, listen to your heart through a stethoscope, and generally test your reflexes.

You should be asked about other medications you are taking. You should be asked about your eating habits, your weight history, and the amount and frequency of your exercise. You should be asked whether or not you smoke tobacco (it's been estimated that one in six people with

Type 2 diabetes smokes). If you do smoke, according to Irl B. Hirsch, M.D., an associate professor of medicine at the University of Washington School of Medicine in Seattle, your doctor should also urge you at every visit to quit, and discuss methods of quitting and drugs that can help the process. If you're a pregnant woman, you should be asked about problems you might have experienced during pregnancy.

If your doctor skips any of these steps, do something about it. Taking off your shoes and socks before the doctor comes into the room may remind him or her to check your feet. One well-informed woman shyly wiggles her toes if her doctor seems to be forgetting this important step. You can even take a checklist into the office with you if you think your doctor might miss something, although this will probably not be appreciated.

Yes, medical doctors are busy. Please don't waste your doctor's time on irrelevant chatter. But when it's necessary, assert yourself on your own behalf.

YOUR TREATMENT PLAN

By the end of the first visit or series of visits, you should have worked out a diabetes care plan with your health-care team. Your treatment plan should consider you and your lifestyle—your work or travel schedule, your eating preferences, your cultural background, and any other medical problems you might have. You may have met with a nurse practitioner, a diabetes educator, a dietitian, or other members of your health-care team. You may have been given referrals for later appointments, or even had those appointments set up for you. Follow the recommendations your doctor gives you for follow-up appointments. If you happen to miss an appointment, call and set another one.

Although some similarities exist, you are not exactly like every other person who has diabetes. Therefore, your treatment plan should not be the exact same one given to all patients who see your doctor. In some cases, you may have to adapt the plan to yourself. Doing so gives it a much higher chance of success, and gives you more control and participation in the process.

A diabetes care plan is thorough if it includes both short- and long-term goals. The American Diabetes Association recommends that every good diabetes care plan include the following:

- Educational sessions on how to measure blood glucose levels, how to keep records, and how to treat low blood sugar.
- Advice on eating prepared by a dietitian.
- Recommendations on lifestyle changes that you should make, such as doing regular exercise or stopping smoking.
- A written list of medicines that you will use for control (if medicines are prescribed).
- Instructions on when to return to the doctor, and when you should call if you have a question or an emergency.

In addition, your plan should include a referral to visit an eye doctor, a foot doctor, a dentist, and other specialists as needed.

If you are a woman who may wish to have children, a good diabetes care plan will include a birth-control and prepregnancy plan. It's certainly possible to have healthy children if you have diabetes, but planning for pregnancy in advance will give you the best chance for a successful pregnancy and birth. *Gestational diabetes,* or diabetes that occurs during pregnancy, is addressed at length in chapter 12.

FREQUENCY OF VISITS

As a rule of thumb, the better your health, the less you will need to see your doctor. Two or three doctor visits per year are sufficient if you have no complications and have good glucose control.

Your doctor may want you to come back or call in more frequently in certain situations, such as when you are making major changes in your diabetes care plan. If you are having trouble controlling your glucose levels, or just beginning insulin or other medications, you should see your doctor at least four times per year.

The American Diabetes Association recommends that all follow-up visits to the doctor who is managing your diabetes should include the following:

- Measuring weight and blood pressure.
- Examining your eyes and feet.
- Asking to see your blood glucose records.
- Taking blood for a glycosylated hemoglobin test, and urine for a urine test.
- An inquiry about problems you've had since the last visit, such as other illnesses or other life problems.
- Asking what adjustments you've made to your plan.
- Asking about problems you're having in following your plan.
- Asking about incidences of high or low blood sugar.
- Asking about symptoms of possible complications.
- A review of your treatment plan to measure progress and identify problem areas.

In addition to the doctor who treats your diabetes, you may have a *primary care physician,* typically a doctor of internal medicine or family practitioner, who oversees your basic health care. These general practitioners were once called family doctors. Ideally, your primary care physician should understand diabetes, and know when to refer you to a specialist. In some cases, the primary care physician can be the primary medical manager of your diabetes, and use diabetologists or endocrinologists only as consultants in your care. It is estimated that 80 percent of the people with diabetes in the United States are under the care of a

FREQUENCY OF VISITS

Here are some generally accepted guidelines regarding frequency of visits to doctors and other specialists. These recommendations may vary from person to person, depending on their physical condition and the recommendations of their personal physician.

More than once a year:

- The medical doctor who is treating your diabetes should be seen at least twice a year, and at least four times per year if you are using insulin.
- A foot specialist, called a podiatrist or an orthopedist, should be seen every six months.
- A dentist or periodontist should be seen every six months.

At least once a year:

- Primary care physician
- Ophthalmologist or eye doctor
- Nurse educator or certified diabetes educator
- Registered dietitian or nutritionist
- Exercise physiologist

On an as-needed basis:

- Mental health professionals
- Other medical specialists
- Support groups

primary care physician, while only about 20 percent are under the care of an endocrinologist. The doctor who treats your diabetes is important. In 1999, a survey printed in *Diabetes Care* stated that the number one cause of poor diabetes care was the doctor.

COMMUNICATION

Communicating with your doctor and your health-care team is important. It's your responsibility to alert them to your problems since they cannot read your mind or anticipate every situation that might come up. Since these people are often in a hurry, some planning will assure that your most important questions are answered. Polite assertiveness is often helpful. When asking questions, ask the doctor to repeat any answers that you don't understand the first time. If you have a lot of questions, notify your doctor's office beforehand so that the receptionist can try to schedule extra time for you with the doctor.

To make sure that you get your most important questions answered, you may approach a visit to your doctor as something like a business meeting. Experts on doctor-patient communication suggest the following steps to deal with a meeting with your doctor, steps that could easily apply to meetings with any health-care professional:

- Write down a few questions in advance.
- Mail, fax, or deliver a copy of your questions to the doctor before going in to see him or her.
- After your doctor has examined you, go down your list of questions, one at a time, and get your questions answered.
- Write down or tape-record the doctor's answers so that you will remember them.
- Repeat what the doctor said back to him or her before you leave the office, so that the doctor can correct any misunderstandings right away.

Diabetes treatment takes time, particularly at first, when you are educating yourself about your own care. Some health-care organizations, hospitals, and clinics have very good educational programs, and you should avail yourself of these whenever possible.

If you are having a lot of trouble in the early stages of your diabetes, it may be possible for you to visit one of the major diabetes clinics and stay for a few days while you are examined and given various tests. Some of these clinics have excellent educational programs and classes that will teach you the basics of good self-care in a comfortable setting.

Your health-care team includes specialists who all have roles to play in your treatment. As you learn their roles, you will learn who to ask about what. For instance, the registered dietitian or nutritionist is probably the best person to ask if you are having trouble changing your eating patterns or are reacting to a particular food. And a mental health professional is probably the best person to see if your diagnosis or prognosis is causing you to have serious problems overcoming such emotions as anger, depression, or fear.

In this partnership approach, it's your job to notify your doctor or nurse if your blood sugar is unusually high, if you have symptoms you don't understand, if a particular medication is not working as expected, or any other time you experience significant problems. Given the current state of the medical system, you may have to speak up for yourself if you don't get the services you are entitled to receive.

Many problems may be solved with a phone call rather than a doctor's visit. Before you have medical problems at home, ask your doctor or nurse when the best time is to call with questions. When you do call, ask when you may expect to receive a response. Some doctors set aside a certain time of day to return calls, and asking about a doctor's schedule may save you some time sitting by the telephone, waiting for a return call.

When you do see a new doctor, bring a list of the medications you currently take—including each drug's name, the quantity you take, the number of times you take it, and how you are taking it if it's different from the manner prescribed. Your new doctor will probably want to see your previous doctor's charts, test results, lab reports, and imaging studies such as X rays. You can contact your old doctor and request copies of these things, allowing adequate time to copy and assemble them, and then pick them up in person and deliver them to your new doctor either in person or by mail with a cover letter.

Remember that nobody has a greater stake in your good health than you. Consider yourself an important member of your health-care team. You're not the medical expert or the exercise expert or the diet expert, but you're the world expert on you. Know your rights, as recommended by the American Diabetes Association, and insist upon good medical care from your doctors. Don't be obnoxious or abusive to people who are trying to help you, but assert yourself when necessary. If you need to blow a trumpet in the examining room to get a nagging question answered, blow that trumpet, because sometimes asserting yourself is the only way to catch the attention of a busy medical professional.

It can be quite empowering to educate yourself about diabetes, and to develop a treatment plan with your doctor and the other specialists on your medical team. Know your medical treatment rights, as outlined by the American Diabetes Association, and make sure those treatment recommendations are followed. As the next chapter explains, diabetes involves a set of known biological facts that can be understood. You can put this information to good use in the management of your diabetes.

Chapter 4

BIOLOGY

How Diabetes Develops and Affects the Human Body

$\sim$

THIS CHAPTER EXPLAINS HOW DIABETES CAN AFFECT THE HUMAN BODY. WHEN YOU HAVE diabetes, your normal metabolism is slightly thrown off. The most crucial relationship in diabetes is the one between a digested sugar, called glucose, and the essential hormone, insulin. There are several ways in which high levels of glucose can affect the normal actions of the human body. If you understand these effects, your treatment will make more sense.

A diagnosis of diabetes is a call to action. A fasting plasma glucose (FPG) reading of greater than 126 mg/dl or 7.0 mmol/L after fasting (eating nothing and drinking only water for eight hours prior to the test) is the current standard for diagnosing diabetes, according to clinical practice guidelines released by the ADA in 1999. Glucose above 200 mg/dl (11.1 mmol/L) with symptoms of diabetes, after two hours of an oral glucose tolerance test, also confirms a diagnosis of diabetes. A random glucose reading of greater than 160 mg/dl (or 8.9 mmol/L) at any time is considered a positive screening result, but a diagnosis of diabetes should be confirmed by further testing. The glycosylated hemoglobin test is also used to diagnose diabetes. Another test, the C-peptide test, measures approximately how much insulin your body produces. Although some doctors still use the term *borderline diabetes,* the current thinking is that no such thing as borderline diabetes actually exists. In short, you either have diabetes or you don't. If you have it, it should be treated.

Diabetes is a disease that creates a continual problem with the way in which the body utilizes food. The breakdown of food is a part of the constant ebb and flow of food and energy within your body, a process called *metabolism.* In people with diabetes, the body digests food normally, but the nutrients that pass into the bloodstream cannot be properly utilized by the body's cells.

GENESIS OF MAN

Diabetes has been around for a long time. Around 1500 B.C., medical scribes in both Egypt and India mentioned a disease characterized by great thirst and the passing of great amounts of sugary urine. The relationship between diabetes and sugar in the human diet was recognized early on, and many early treatment attempts involved limiting the dietary intake of sugar and sweets. One treatment recommended in India three thousand years ago involved strenuous exercise.

Although physicians have diagnosed diabetes for thousands of years, they have only recently begun to understand how to treat it. For many years, people with diabetes could expect to live foreshortened lives. A standard estimate of life expectancy for people with diabetes was that, all things being equal, diabetes could shorten human life by as much as one-third.

Why do human beings get diabetes? For almost two million years, anthropologists tell us, our primitive ancestors roamed the earth trying to keep themselves alive in a hostile world by hunting and gathering food. Huge amounts of physical energy were burned away just staying alive in a world without fast food, TV sets, automobiles, or central heating and air-conditioning.

The meat consumed by our ancestors came from free-roaming wild animals, whose bodies contained a much lower percentage of fat than domesticated animals, whose activities are restricted. Fish had to be caught, antelope hunted, eggs found and gathered, edible plants located and picked, all with a constant expenditure of physical energy. For tens of thousands of generations, our ancestors exhausted the food sources in one area, then abruptly moved on. To endure this harsh, primitive lifestyle, the humans who lived long enough to reproduce were those whose bodies could hoard enough nutrients to keep them alive, sometimes for long periods of time, between meals.

Civilization as we know it has lasted less than 1 percent as long as the hunter-gatherer phase of human existence, which became defunct only with the invention of agriculture just a few hundred generations ago. Considering the period of time in which human beings have roamed the earth, all human history since the Renaissance is merely a wink in time. Evolution is slow; human anatomy hasn't changed much over the past few centuries. We no longer need periodic bursts of great physical strength, or to retain nutrients in our bodies for long periods of time. Consequently, great numbers of people get fat and flabby. And many of us get Type 2 diabetes, a disease strongly associated with obesity and a lack of physical exercise.

THE BIOLOGY OF DIABETES

To understand the biology of diabetes, think of the human body as a series of interlocking systems that work together to keep us alive. The circulatory, respiratory, and digestive systems all must work together for the body to be able to utilize food. The circulatory system, consisting of the heart and many miles of blood vessels, continually circulates blood past the digestive tract and the lungs, back and forth to every part of your body, making a complete circuit approximately every twenty seconds. Your respiratory system, which includes your lungs, continually huffs and puffs in oxygen from the air, and pumps it into the bloodstream. When you eat, food goes through the gastrointestinal, or digestive, system, where your stomach breaks down food into tiny digestible bits. These molecules of food move through your intestines into your bloodstream, where they accompany the oxygen in your red blood cells to the furthest reaches of your body to provide energy and fuel for your cells.

Much of the food we eat is broken down into a simple sugar called *glucose,* the most important carbohydrate in our metabolism. Since glucose is oxidized and used directly by the brain and nervous system, we must *always* have some in our bloodstream. Normally comprising approximately one-tenth of 1 percent of our blood (roughly equivalent to a spoonful of sugar), glucose is a vital substance, but problems occur when too much or too little of it is held in the blood.

After we eat, the amount of glucose in our bloodstream temporarily rises until it is absorbed to provide energy and nourishment. When diabetes is present, glucose *cannot* be properly absorbed by the cells. Consequently, glucose levels rise. This backup of glucose in the blood damages the body. Excessive glucose levels, called *high blood sugar,* are a continuing health risk for every person with diabetes, and must be controlled.

GLUCOSE AND INSULIN

In the bodies of most people, glucose is absorbed into the cells with the aid of an essential hormone, *insulin,* the only hormone in the body that lowers blood sugar. Insulin is produced in a gland called the *pancreas,* one of several glands in the endocrine system. Located just behind and below the stomach, the pancreas is about the size of a tennis ball, and weighs about 1 pound. Insulin is secreted from a group of cells hanging off the pancreas like a sort of tail, the *islets of Langerhans.* Insulin is normally secreted by the pancreas every time we need it, in perfectly timed and perfectly measured amounts. A first phase insulin response begins almost immediately, within ten minutes of eating. Insulin's presence helps the tiny particles of glucose move from the red blood cells into the cells of our body, a process that nourishes us and sustains life.

Insulin is a crucial hormone for people with diabetes, whether they

---

DAMAGE BY EXCESSIVE GLUCOSE

With the exception of the brain, the organs of the body most likely to be damaged by diabetes are those that do not require the presence of insulin to metabolize blood glucose.

Can be damaged:

- Eyes
- Kidneys
- Nerves
- Blood vessels

Generally not damaged:

- Brain
- Liver
- Muscles

---

are Type 1 or Type 2. Insulin is most necessary for people with Type 1 diabetes. Type 1 diabetes, once known as juvenile onset diabetes, is sometimes called *insulin dependent diabetes mellitus,* or IDDM. People with Type 1 diabetes don't produce any insulin in their bodies; because they can't metabolize glucose, it backs up in their blood in life-threatening amounts. People with Type 1 diabetes must have insulin injections for their bodies to utilize glucose, and they often must fight simply to retain a healthy weight.

The insulin story is more complex in Type 2 diabetes. Type 2 diabetes, the most common form of diabetes, was once known as maturity onset diabetes because it most frequently appears in older people. Since insulin is not necessary to sustain life, Type 2 diabetes is also known as *non-insulin-dependent diabetes mellitus,* or NIDDM. In Type 2 diabetes, the body produces insulin, often in excessive amounts. However, the insulin actually produced is inadequate to normalize the levels of blood sugar. This occurs because the person with Type 2 diabetes does not produce adequate levels of insulin or his body has become resistant to insulin's effects, a condition called *insulin resistance.* People with Type 2 diabetes who have insulin resistance often produce more than enough insulin within their bodies, and they are frequently overweight.

For people with Type 2 diabetes, the metabolic effects of the disease are not sudden and can be difficult to spot. Compared to Type 1 diabetes, Type 2 diabetes is a much less dramatic disease, a tortoise compared to a hare. The glacial pace with which Type 2 diabetes appears is part of the problem, since treatment cannot begin until diabetes is actually diagnosed.

Type 2 diabetes is generally defined as an impairment of metabolism associated with insulin resistance and an insufficiency of insulin production to compensate for the resistance. All people with Type 2 diabetes produce some insulin. In fact, most produce more than enough insulin when they are diagnosed; these people can often control their diabetes with disciplined lifestyle changes. However, about one in every six people with Type 2 diabetes has a pancreas that does not produce enough insulin to metabolize the available glucose. This small group benefits from lifestyle changes, but they must also take medication to stimulate insulin production, or take supplemental insulin.

Approximately 88 percent of Type 2 diabetics are overweight, and excessive insulin production is a factor. The appetites of these individuals are actually *stimulated* by the excess insulin, causing them to eat more. Overeating and excessive weight gain may actually be caused by a condition called *hyperinsulinemia,* a result of too much insulin in the blood. In addition to its important role in metabolism, insulin also helps the body hold fats by inhibiting the hormones that break them down.

THE IMPORTANCE OF INSULIN

In Victorian times, research scientists seeking the cause of diabetes honed in on the pancreas, a comma-shaped gland located behind and beneath the stomach. In 1921, insulin was discovered. Before long, commercial insulin was given to human beings, allowing a measure of control over diabetes. In the 1950s, medical researchers discovered the resistance to insulin at the cellular level that is characteristic of Type 2 diabetes. This allowed Type 2 diabetes to be precisely identified as a related but distinct form of diabetes, which could be approached and treated in a different way.

Insulin is secreted by the pancreas of the average person at a rate of approximately 20 to 30 units per day in rhythmic pulses perfectly timed with the absorption of food. Insulin chemically accompanies glucose into the cells of your body, where glucose combines with oxygen to produce energy, then breaks down into carbon dioxide and water. Insulin helps convert glucose into fats called triglycerides. Insulin also helps convert glucose into another form of sugar called glycogen, which is stored in the body for emergency use.

A lack of insulin (or insulin ineffectively used) throws off the natural balance of the body, known as *homeostasis*. Trying to maintain homeostasis without proper insulin is a bit like trying to win a football game without a quarterback. The absorption of glucose into the body is continually blocked in people with Type 2 diabetes, even though the necessary elements, glucose and insulin, are present, sometimes in excessive amounts.

For many years, researchers believed that fat cells somehow impeded the ability of this insulin to "open the door" to each cell's absorption of glucose. The current thinking is that a chemical substance produced in fat tissue, called the *tumor necrosis factor alpha,* is somehow transferred from fat cells to muscle cells, thereby impairing the normally ravenous consumption of glucose by the muscles. Another hormone produced in the pancreas, glucagon, normally has a counterbalancing effect to insulin, and plays a role in Type 2 diabetes.

Whatever the cause, people with Type 2 diabetes don't utilize all of the glucose created from food. This is a simplified explanation, by necessity, because glucose goes through several chemical processes before it is converted to energy. The human body is a complex but well-orchestrated place in which an estimated six trillion chemical reactions take place every second.

HIGH BLOOD SUGAR

Most people don't even notice the first rise in their blood sugar levels because the backup of glucose in the blood occurs slowly, over many years. At the time that Type 2 diabetes is diagnosed, most people have *very high* blood glucose levels, and steps must be taken immediately to bring down those levels.

In addition to the glucose produced directly from food, more glucose is added to the bloodstream by the liver and other organs that are biologically programmed to release sugar in times of deprivation; this release assures that the brain always has enough glucose to function. The liver typically cranks out extra glucose after you sleep for six or eight hours or when you don't eat, because it gets biochemical signals from your body that glucose isn't getting into your cells. Supplemental glucose production kicks into high gear when you get sick. High blood sugar sometimes occurs during pregnancy and during times of great physical and emotional stress, since adrenalin is one of the five hormones in the body that counters the effects of insulin.

High and low levels of blood sugar do not normally remain in the bloodstream for long because the swift insulin response keeps blood sugar at about 0.1 percent of our blood. Our bodies deal with normal fluctuations of glucose and insulin as a matter of course, but the human body has difficulty with greater fluctuations, particularly with levels that remain high. High blood sugar levels are dangerous because they damage the body over time.

The very high blood sugar levels associated with Type 2 diabetes are not healthy for many reasons. Since your cells can't absorb all of the glucose backed up in the bloodstream, they can be starved for nutrients, even with high levels of glucose nearby. The extra weight carried by many men and women with Type 2 diabetes strains the body in several ways, as high levels of fats clog the blood vessels and raise blood pressure. High levels of glucose can actually nourish the bacteria that cause infections inside the body, and glucose can inhibit the normal infection-fighting abilities of white blood cells; both of these factors slow down the rate of healing and compromise the immune system. Two other harmful effects of high blood sugar levels are *protein glycosylation* and *oxidation,* which occur at the cellular and molecular levels, too small to ever be seen by the naked eye.

GLYCOSYLATION

When blood sugar levels are high, small, simple blood sugar molecules attach themselves to the larger and more complicated protein molecules in the blood, a process called *glycosylation.* A bit of glycosylation occurs in every person, but high blood sugar causes much more of it. Glycosylation creates protein molecules that are damaged; they in turn disable other proteins, called *enzymes,* that are needed in many processes within the body. Glycosylation makes the protein-rich membranes of the red blood cells stiffen, something like partially frozen water balloons. Stiff cell membranes make it difficult for nutrient-carrying red blood cells to squeeze through the body's smallest blood vessels, which can cause the vessels to rupture. Stiffened red blood cells scrape against and slightly scar the walls of larger blood vessels, making the blood vessel walls stiffer than normal and forming shallow pockets that trap fatty substances such as cholesterol. These factors can raise the blood pressure and increase the risk of heart attack and other complications.

Besides the cell membranes, the eyes, skin, cartilage, and blood vessel walls also need high levels of protein to function properly. These areas are especially compromised by high concentrations of glycosylated proteins. In addition to this damage, glycosylated proteins may also link together, forming harmful cross-linked biochemical products known as *advanced glycosylation end-products,* or AGEs. Among other things, these end-products may contribute to the aging process. Fortunately, excess glycosylation may be slowed down or halted with good blood sugar control.

The normal process of *oxidation* is impaired by diabetes. Within the cells, oxygen is used to convert substances such as glucose into energy. Unfortunately, about 2 percent of the body's available oxygen causes trouble by converting into "free radicals." These chemically unstable molecules set off small but ultimately harmful molecular chain reactions that damage the molecular structure of other cells. Free radicals are believed to contribute to cancer, brain damage, and possibly to severe insulin reactions, according to health writer John Walsh. Free radicals are believed to initiate the process that ends with the creation of AGEs. As these damaging chemical processes occur, beneficial chemical substances called *antioxidants* can disable free radicals, and restore chemical stability to wild, unstable cells. Unfortunately, levels of antioxidant vitamins, such as vitamin C and vitamin E, are often lower than normal in the bloodstreams of people with diabetes.

Taking positive steps to lower your blood sugar level will contribute to your health, even within the molecular depths of your body, because lower blood sugar will help you properly utilize food and inhibit potential damage from glycosylation and oxidation.

A disciplined combination of healthy eating and a vigorous, healthy lifestyle helps control diabetes in many people. One physician estimates that most people with Type 2 diabetes should be able to control their disease for twenty to thirty years using lifestyle changes alone, if their blood sugars have not been out of whack for too long.

Diabetes is a disease of the metabolism—something goes wrong with the way in which the body utilizes food. Its roots are deep in human history. The hormone insulin plays a key role in helping the body to metabolize glucose, a simple but important form of sugar found in the blood. The high blood glucose levels that result from Type 2 diabetes can damage the body in many ways over time. The good news is that you have the power to lower and control your own blood sugar level in a number of ways, including the use of self-management and stress-management techniques, both of which are explained in the next chapter.

Chapter 5

SELF-MANAGEMENT

Managing Negative Stress Helps You Manage Diabetes

~

SELF-MANAGEMENT IS A PROCESS OF LEARNING AND APPLYING NEW KNOWLEDGE. What you will need to achieve good self-management are a few basic tools. These include changes in lifestyle, medications, and self-testing on a regular basis. Since having diabetes can be extremely stressful, one of the first aspects of self-management that you can integrate into your life may well be stress management, an aspect highlighted in this chapter.

"It is by the presence of mind in untried emergencies that the native mettle of a man is tested," wrote American poet and essayist James Russell Lowell. Joseph Califano, former secretary of health, education, and welfare, observed, "You, the individual, can do more for your health and well-being than any doctor, any hospital, any drug, and any exotic medical device."

Both of these remarks apply to diabetes. The self-management of diabetes involves learning to act on your own behalf. A program of good self-management will help you feel physically and emotionally better in the short run, improve the overall quality of your life, and keep you as healthy as possible in the years ahead. How far you take this concept is up to you.

Self-management primarily involves educating yourself, monitoring your medical condition, and working with your health-care team to adopt lifestyle changes. Self-management may also involve an effort to combat negative or excessive stress, something you can influence and control.

Sisyphus spent his life trying to push a huge boulder up a hill, only to have it roll down again. Self-management doesn't have to feel like that kind of impossible, unending task. For the first few weeks, as you educate yourself, self-management will take time and energy. It may frustrate you. It may seem endless. You may well feel like Sisyphus, as familiar routines are broken and new responsibilities are assumed. In the beginning, you may feel that you'll *never* get a break from diabetes. After all, self-management basically involves exercising some discipline over our indulgences, those bedeviling urges and impulses to which we have so often abandoned ourselves.

Believe it or not, you can integrate self-management into your life. Many of the things you'll do may become as routine as finding a few minutes each day to comb your hair or brush or floss your teeth. After all, you don't resent that you must brush your teeth every time you pick up your toothbrush—you just do it. As the following story demonstrates, good self-management involves learning what to do, and then applying that knowledge to your life.

STEVE'S STORY

A successful sales manager, whom we shall call Steve, took quick effective steps to bring his diabetes under control within a year, something he achieved with the help of a supportive wife and a good medical doctor.

A former college quarterback, fifty-three-year-old Steve had risen through the ranks of a large company to become a regional sales manager, supervising people in several states and traveling frequently. His job challenged him, but he enjoyed it.

A few weeks after he got married for the second time, Steve began having troubling physical symptoms. He unexplainably gained weight and experienced bouts of dry mouth and blurry vision. He went to his doctor for tests. Although he felt fine at the time, Steve's blood glucose level tested extremely high, above 600 mg/dl. He was told that he was "borderline diabetic."

The first thing Steve did was to sit down with his doctor and his new wife and ask what he could do about his high blood sugar. Then, he says, he began "attacking it very aggressively."

His doctor, an internist with many patients who have diabetes, prescribed Glucotrol. He told Steve about an educational program offered through a hospital in a nearby town. Steve and his wife attended the classes and read books about diabetes. Steve joined the American Diabetes Association and searched the Internet for medical information. He bought a glucose meter, began blood testing, and started a daily exercise program. Although he didn't smoke and only occasionally drank, Steve worked to change his diet, too.

"We just did what the books suggested, such as eating smaller portions of certain foods," he says. "Right now, we eat very little meat. We eat a lot of fish, chicken, turkey, fruits and vegetables, and grains and cereals."

Steve has already lost 30 pounds. His exercise program is a daily one-hour walk, which he takes before dinner, sometimes accompanied by his wife, and sometimes walking his dog. He takes a brisk stroll of 3 to 4 miles around the suburban neighborhood where he lives. He walks in a good pair of Reebok walking shoes, and checks his feet every day to make sure that they are fine before he exercises.

"Walking before dinner is a good time for me because it helps me shake off the minor stresses of the day," Steve says. "It also helps me because I'm less hungry after I exercise. My wife is buffing up too. This has helped bring us together as newlyweds."

After less than three months of aggressively combating his high blood sugar, Steve's blood glucose level has fallen to between 75 and 100 mg/dl. He has another 10 pounds to go in achieving his weight-loss goal, but his blurry vision has gone away. His cholesterol level has fallen from a high of about 400 to 239 at his last test. Steve's doctor recently took him off the diabetes medication, which was no longer necessary because his blood sugar level was under control. Steve is almost a textbook case of what people with Type 2 diabetes can do to educate and help themselves.

"My wife and I got into a positive frame of mind on this thing, and decided that we could take control of it," Steve says. "If you want to be successful in life you've got to set goals. I encourage people I work with to do that, and it carries all through my life. I'm a positive thinker. I don't dwell on the negative, and I don't have friends who dwell on negative things. If you know you have a situation, you just go out and take control of it. After all, you've only got one life. You might as well go for it, if you want to live that life well."

FIVE CONCEPTS OF SELF-MANAGEMENT

Good self-management of diabetes uses five general concepts. These five tools are:

- Blood sugar testing
- Nutrition
- Physical activity
- Medication
- Stress management

Each of these concepts may be foreign to you now, but your medical team can help educate you. You can build on this basic information to learn a few things on your own.

The five aspects of self-management may seem bewildering, particularly at first, when it seems like as soon as one question is answered, two more questions pop up in its place. You will soon realize that all five concepts are important, but you may not know which one to put first, which you may let slide, or exactly how much time to devote to one or another. This may be confusing. You may feel like a person who has never juggled suddenly being pushed onto a stage and told to keep four or five balls in the air. You don't have to learn it all right away, but applying some of what you know every day is important. Good self-management involves a judicious use of these five tools, which you will learn about and then utilize in your own way.

Give yourself a period of time, perhaps a month, to begin the process. Learn at your own pace. Integrate what you learn into your own life—one thing at a time if that suits you, or in one grand swoop if that's more your style. Do not force yourself to move faster than you possibly can. Apply what you learn at a comfortable pace, but continue moving forward a little bit each day. The important thing is that you learn eventually, and that you use what you know on your own behalf.

One aspect of self-management that is linked to all the others is blood sugar testing. Your medical team will instruct you in simple home testing techniques that you can use to check your blood sugar levels, and help you to set reasonable blood sugar goals. As will be explained in chapter 6, the blood sugar levels that people with Type 2 diabetes strive to achieve may be a bit above normal, but they are adequate to prevent damage to your health.

Nutrition, dealt with in chapter 7, involves creating a new style of eating that focuses on healthy foods in reasonable quantities. A good eating style should include regular meals that are spaced out, with regular small snacks in between. The adjustments you make, perhaps with the help of a registered dietitian or a nutritional consultant, should be suited to the lifestyle you already have, and your need to control your weight. Any changes in eating style should be reasonable and attainable within the framework of your life.

Adopting a more physically active lifestyle, as explained in chapter 8, is something that will benefit you immediately and over the long term. In conjunction with your doctor, an exercise physiologist, a personal trainer, or perhaps on your own, the changes you make in this area of your life should also mesh well with your lifestyle.

The medications prescribed by the doctor who treats your diabetes, as explained in chapter 9, are a fourth important aspect of your self-management strategy. Although medications are not always used to treat Type 2 diabetes, they should be employed as needed, to bring immediate benefits that outweigh the risks.

Stress management, dealt with in the pages that follow, is another important aspect of self-management, and perhaps the most easily undertaken because it is entirely under your control. Managing negative stress uses methods or techniques that you select to benefit yourself. Stress relief is useful to all people, particularly those with diabetes, because stress raises blood glucose levels, which harm the body over time.

Taken together, this is your tool set for self-management. By educating yourself, by practicing what you learn, and by seeking good medical advice from your medical team when you need it, you can manage diabetes, one day at a time.

"A LONG SORROW"

Physicians have known for years that physical trauma, such as surgery or illness, can affect people with diabetes, greatly elevating their blood sugar levels. Emotional stress also has an obvious relationship with diabetes. As early as 1684, a doctor in Shakespeare's time observed that diabetes was due to "a long sorrow."

The emotional and psychological trauma of negative stress, sometimes called *distress,* may be treated by several methods, including education and psychological counseling. But the medical community's longtime awareness of the ill effects of stress doesn't lead most doctors to recommend particular methods of stress relief, perhaps because this is out of the realm of their expertise. The selection of techniques to relieve stress is also somewhat personal.

Incidents of acute stress affect your body quite rapidly, and in measurable ways. Four hormones, including adrenaline, jump into your bloodstream in a fraction of a second. The release of stress hormones speeds up your metabolism, makes your heart beat faster and pump more blood, and slightly raises your blood pressure. Stress hormones in the bloodstream increase the rate of breathing, begin shutting down the digestive system to divert blood to the muscles, dilate the eyes, heighten hearing, slightly shrink the sex organs, and constrict the arteries in your arms and legs. Stored glucose is released from the liver and muscles, and blood sugar shoots up. Some people with diabetes say this stress-induced adrenaline rush first resembles the symptoms of out-of-control blood sugar—immediate weakness, shakiness, an escalated fast-beating pulse—that returns to normal as glucose is released into the blood. This so-called fight or flight reflex, caused by acute stress, prepares the body for strenuous physical action—struggling with a tiger, perhaps, or running for one's life.

DIABETES IS STRESSFUL

Having diabetes is stressful too. For one thing, there is a built-in high level of stress in the demands of coping with an invisible, chronic, ever-present disease. Diabetes takes time and energy to understand, and it can be difficult to manage. Diabetes can strain a family's finances, or knock retirement plans askew. In addition to that, the ever-present threat of complications hangs over the heads of many people with diabetes, creating more worry and distress. In the 1950s, researchers first noticed a rise in both blood glucose levels and ketone levels in men and women with diabetes who were merely exposed to *conversations* about areas of stress in their lives.

The stress associated with diabetes may become *acute* or temporarily intense at certain times, such as immediately after your diagnosis of diabetes or when you experience complications. But most of the time diabetes is a constant *chronic* stress that lingers in the mind. Chronic stress is chemically and emotionally different than acute stress, which can be more rapidly resolved.

In chronically stressful situations, a steroid hormone called cortisol is released over a period ranging from several minutes to a few hours. Similar to adrenaline, cortisol causes the blood pressure to rise and the pulse rate to slow. Among cortisol's measurable physical effects, the number of white blood cells in your body drops a bit, slightly depressing your immune system. Some amino acids (a form of digested protein) actually change into sugar, or glucose. Other hormones that can be released by stress include growth hormones, thyroid-stimulating hormones, and glucagon. All of these hormones elevate blood glucose.

Chronic stress is constant and primarily emotional, like many of the stresses of modern life. When you live with an excessive level of chronic stress, you must seek ways to reduce it or face the perils of physical or mental exhaustion. When you add diabetes to this mix, negative stress can further elevate your blood glucose and wreak great havoc on your body.

The emotional stresses unique to people with diabetes include the "invisible" and chronic nature of the disease, the frustrations you may experience in trying to control the many variables that can affect blood

HOW STRESS WORKS

The general adaptation syndrome is the way in which physical stress affects the body, according to Hans Selye, M.D., a pioneering researcher in this field. For purposes of simplification, we use a beast in the jungle as the stressor, although the stressor can actually be something as small as a virus or bacteria entering your body, in which case this drama would be played out in miniature through an immune response. If this could be metaphorically extended to the national scale, the general adaptation syndrome would look something like war and peace.

ALARM PHASE—A person sees the beast in the jungle. Biochemical alarms prepare the body. The brain perceives the danger, sending electrical messages down the nerves while hormones such as adrenaline shoot out into the bloodstream. The breath quickens, the muscles tense, the body prepares for "fight or flight" with a quick burst of temporary strength.

RESISTANCE PHASE—You respond to the beast in the jungle by resisting its apparent intention to harm you. You may turn tail and rapidly take flight, or pick up a club and defend yourself. Both alternatives utilize the new supply of stress-induced physical and mental energy.

EXHAUSTION PHASE—You may have run as far away as you possibly could, or fought the beast to the point of exhaustion. Your body has given everything it can to adapt to the stress of meeting the beast, and can give no more.

sugar, and even the very unpredictability of the disease itself. Diabetes puts physical stress on your body, as does a lack of exercise or excess weight. Stress alone may throw off your normal routine of self-management, creating more stress when something as simple as missing a meal or not exercising throws your metabolism for a loop.

Although you probably had diabetes for quite a while before you were actually diagnosed, the idea of having a chronic disease may have hit you hard. For some, a diagnosis of diabetes is up there with life's most stressful and emotionally upsetting events, such as the death of a spouse, divorce, a jail term, or being fired from a job.

The stress of having diabetes may be compounded by what at first seems to be a *huge* amount of information that you are asked to master to keep your diabetes in control. Even small variations between your goals and your first efforts at control may set you off, frustrate you, or vex you.

"For me, the anxiety of being new to diabetes seemed to affect my *intelligence,*" one well-spoken woman in her forties confessed. "For instance, once when I was trying to write a note, I couldn't even write the word *sure.* I had to cross out that word three or four times before I got it right. Then I saw a headline in the newspaper that read Panacea Cure, but I read it as Pancreas Cure, which was where my mind was. I got to the point where my own anxiety was scaring me."

The first few weeks can be a very stressful time for not only the person diagnosed, but also for loved ones. Life goals and future expectations may have to be revised. Accepting changes can be a painful process for any family, as chapter 13 explains.

It's certainly an adjustment to move into the maintenance phase of self-management, with all the required learning and changes to lifestyle. But it is an adjustment that millions of people all over the world have made.

"I've had to learn to control the *outside* factors in my life to manage stress," a woman told her support group. "The other day I had two major events to attend; I knew both would be very stressful. I chose to attend only one event because I knew I couldn't attend them both. I've had to learn to make these choices since I was diagnosed with diabetes, to keep my blood sugar in control."

Stress may contribute to either excessive weight loss or weight gain. Hans Selye, M.D., observed some years ago in The Stress of Life that "excessive obesity may also be a manifestation of stress, especially in people with certain types of frustrating mental experiences. A person who does not get enough satisfaction from work or from his relations with other people may be driven to find consolation in almost anything that may provide comfort." Even though the predisposition toward diabetes is inherited, Dr. Selye stated, "It depends largely upon the way the body reacts to stress whether or not a latent diabetic tendency will develop into a manifest disease." He noted that in some cases diabetes does not spring from an insufficient production of insulin, but from an overproduction of stress-related hormones that raise the blood sugar.

Stress contributes to fatigue, as does high blood sugar, poor nutrition, dehydration, lack of exercise, and smoking. Stress is known to deplete the body of stores of certain necessary vitamins, such as vitamin C and the B vitamins. Among its other ill effects, stress depletes the body of a necessary chemical called serotonin, most of which is manufactured in the body during deep sleep. Serotonin depletion leads to carbohydrate cravings, making it more difficult to maintain a program of healthy eating and to lose weight, according to Los Angeles endocrinologist Calvin Ezrin, M.D. Whether or not you have diabetes, it's important to recognize and control stress.

If worrying about diabetes has affected your sleeping patterns or your normal weight, or has resulted in great changes in your moods, these are signs of depression or anxiety that should be treated by a psychiatrist, psychologist, or other mental health professional.

STRESS MANAGEMENT TECHNIQUES

Fortunately, you may learn to avoid or manage stress by using any number of safe, sensible techniques. All of these may be enjoyable, and some are quite inexpensive. A few may already be part of your program of self-management. Some may be practiced a few minutes at a time, at work or at home. A few are best learned from expert instructors in formal classes or in groups. Some may enhance your social life. The bottom line is to find stress-relieving techniques that suit and benefit you.

Remember that reducing stress will help you control diabetes because lowering stress can help reduce dangerously high glucose levels. Beginning a program of stress management will give you more control over your life. Fortunately, it's quite safe to experiment with any of the stress-relieving techniques listed below. If you need a further inducement to control excessive stress, research has begun to show that relieving stress can beef up your immune system, and decrease the likelihood of contracting other health problems such as heart disease, mental illness, and cancer.

Positive ways of coping with stress include modifying your own behavior, exercise, good eating habits, meditation, biofeedback, distraction, relaxation techniques, counseling, support groups, and even prayer. Negative ways of dealing with stress include drinking, smoking, overeating, skipping meals, isolation, internalizing feelings, abuse of family or friends, and skipping doctor's appointments. Avoid all negative ways of dealing with stress because they actually add to your stress levels by depleting you physically and/or mentally.

Even if you are lucky enough to have a doctor who is knowledgeable about the latest breakthroughs in diabetes care, or if you have vowed to teach yourself more about managing diabetes, education is one of the most powerful tools you have to help alleviate stress and make your life more comfortable and satisfying. Education is the first step toward improving the quality of your life.

Methods that can relieve stress are numerous, and they are not all listed here. Some stress-relieving activities or techniques that work for many people include the following:

CHANGING YOUR BEHAVIOR

You have two ways of changing your behavior to deal with stress that you can anticipate. The first is to avoid the stressful person or situation, the second is to take steps to minimize the effects of stress on you. Many times, you can reduce stress by planning ahead and taking steps to avoid situations or people that you *know* will be stressful. For example, if Uncle Jerry always ropes you into a heated political argument during the family dinner, ask your hostess not to seat you next to him. Or if Uncle Jerry tries to bait you into an argument from across the room, simply don't participate. If driving in rush hour traffic is very stressful for you, perhaps you can arrange to travel at a time of day when traffic isn't so bad, get a cellular telephone in your car to call ahead if you're going to be late, or just hop in a taxi or bus. Make an effort to not let petty annoyances get blown up into major frustrations. When you invest a big part of yourself in the outcome of a particular event or in the behavior of another person, you give that event or that person a measure of power over your life. By trimming your personal investment in troublesome areas, your own behavior may help you achieve a measure of control over predictable stress.

If you have been fretting and worrying over a particular personal or business problem, it may relieve stress to simply deal with that problem. For instance, if you worry that your family will break apart in a bitter fight over your property after you die, call a lawyer and make a will that divides your assets in a way that is fair to everyone concerned.

Here is a useful tool to help you sort out what is—and is not—controllable in your life. It's called the Serenity Prayer, and it's often employed by twelve-step programs all over the world.

THE SERENITY PRAYER

God grant me the serenity
To accept the things I cannot change
The courage to change the things that I can,
And the wisdom to know the difference.

Written by world-famous theologian Reinhold Niebuhr, the Serenity Prayer points out in a simple, concise way that some aspects of your life are simply not within your control, and others are. That you have diabetes is a thing you cannot change. On the other hand, you can find the courage to make changes in the way you live your life, changes of lifestyle that will help you manage and control your diabetes.

EXERCISE

Remember that the fight or flight reflex that accompanies acute distress discharges chemicals such as adrenaline into your blood system. These chemicals prepare your body for physical action—in primitive times, this reflex helped our ancestors to choose between grappling with a beast in the jungle or sprinting to safety. Consequently, it's probably no surprise to learn that a natural way to relieve stress is to get some exercise. Even a quiet walk around the block when you feel stressed out will probably make you feel better. The benefits of exercise in the self-management of Type 2 diabetes are legendary. Physical activities such as swimming, hiking, skiing, or attending low-impact aerobic exercise classes will help you throw off the stress hormones that have swamped your bloodstream. Setting aside a particular time each day for exercise could help you work more physical activity into your life. An "exercise prescription" will be a part of your diabetes treatment plan, as chapter 8 explains, because exercise produces beneficial chemicals of its own.

GOOD NUTRITION

The stress-relieving effects of good nutrition are subtle, and they don't take effect immediately. Since stress depletes levels of some essential vitamins and minerals from the body, changing your eating style to include very nutritious foods, and perhaps a multivitamin supplement, may help you deal with and recover from stressful events. If you don't believe that food can affect your stress levels, watch a coffee drinker try to stop drinking coffee for two or three days. As chapter 7 explains, eating well-balanced, regular meals and faithfully enjoying a small snack in between will help you avoid the stress that comes with quick, erratic meals and a haphazard, fast-food lifestyle that can cause great fluctuations in blood sugar.

RELAXATION EXERCISES

Deep breathing and relaxation exercises are popular ways to deal with stress, and they don't involve strenuous physical activity. Audiotapes and videotapes that instruct you on how to relax are available at bookstores, libraries, drugstores, and video stores, and through mail-order houses. Most have soothing music in the background, and a pleasant voice instructing you on how to breathe deeply and let your various groups of muscles relax, one group at a time. You can set aside a period of time each day for this, your quiet time. Even a few minutes of relaxation or breathing exercises here and there will help, particularly if you're under immediate stress and need some quick relief—even at work.

MEDITATION

Whether it's the ancient Eastern mode of transcendental meditation or the less formal "relaxation response" popularized by Harvard University physician Herbert Benson, M.D., meditation can help you cope with stress. While physical or emotional stress pumps stress hormones into the body, the relaxation response has a stress-reducing effect. Research has shown that meditation can be useful for many people with Type 2 diabetes, and can help lower blood glucose and blood pressure over time. Meditation has been called the other side of prayer because it is a spiritual activity in which the practitioner does not communicate with a higher power but simply coexists with it.

YOGA

Hatha yoga is an ancient Eastern system of breathing and muscle stretching which combines many of the benefits of deep breathing, meditation, and exercise. A great number of relaxation techniques are spin-offs from yoga. The first written documents of yoga were compiled by a man named Patanjali sometime before the year 300. Legend has it that yoga was passed down orally for many generations, originating perhaps as early as 5000 B.C.

Although the word *yoga* may conjure up images of white-robed, full-bearded religious leaders, it is a superb exercise for most people with diabetes because of its stress-reducing benefits. A study involving people with Type 2 diabetes, published in *Diabetes Research and Clinical Practice* in 1993, found that 104 of the 149 subjects showed a "fair to good" response after practicing yoga for only forty days. Yoga improves balance and flexibility and provides an enhanced sense of well-being because it works all the muscle groups in the body. Yoga is a cornerstone of Dr. Dean Ornish's program for reversing heart disease through lifestyle and diet changes.

Yoga classes are available through schools, senior citizens' centers, the YMCA, the YWCA, and sports clubs. Videos, books, and other materials can assist in practicing yoga at home. The older hatha yoga is a mild form of exercise that combines stretching with frequent intervals of relaxation and deep breathing. Newer, Americanized forms called "power yoga" are quite different, and more akin to aerobic exercise. Discuss yoga or any other exercise program with your doctor before beginning classes.

BIOFEEDBACK

Biofeedback involves simple machines that can help make you aware of your own body. When properly administered, biofeedback will help you relax groups of muscles that are tense, and give you feedback when you succeed. You tell the biofeedback technician what soothes you, then you practice pulling these thoughts into your mind to help relieve your stress. Once you get it down, you can use biofeedback techniques in times of stress. You can even learn to soothe particular groups of muscles. In research studies, more than 80 percent of subjects with Type 2 diabetes used biofeedback to reduce elevated blood glucose levels caused by stress. To find a clinician trained in biofeedback, call the Association for Applied Psychophysiology and Biofeedback, whose address and telephone number are listed in Appendix A, "Other Resources" in the back of this book.

IMAGERY AND VISUALIZATION

Visual imaging techniques were originally developed for the treatment of serious diseases such as cancer to extend the life spans of terminal cancer patients. *Getting Well Again,* by O. Carl Simonton, M.D., Stephanie Matthews-Simonton, and James L. Creighton, is one of the best books on visualization techniques, which may help reduce stress levels and promote healing in people who are chronically ill. Visual imagery is not unlike a system of organized relaxation and daydreaming, in which you regularly place yourself in a quiet relaxed state, then call up mental images that are healthful and beneficial to you. You visualize images targeted to a particular area of your body to help your body heal. You might visualize a flock of descending birds, for instance, as an image to help lower your blood sugar or decrease insulin resistance. Or you might imagine a globe of healing white light descending into your body, to gently stimulate your pancreas to make more insulin. You can learn imagery or visualization techniques in classes or from a book, then utilize them at home.

DISTRACTION

Plug in anything you truly enjoy doing right here. Fishing, shopping, walking the dog, listening to good music, even just watching a good soap opera or baseball game on television—all can distract you by taking your mind off your problems for awhile. Distraction can relieve stress if you've been obsessively worrying about your health and you need to get your mind off your problems. Volunteering to support a cause you believe in or helping another person in need is of great benefit because such actions not only relieve stress but also make you feel less isolated, powerless, and alone. Local offices of the American Diabetes Association and other health organizations often need volunteers.

THINK POSITIVELY

There's accumulating evidence that thinking positively is beneficial for your health. In some research studies, just laughing or forcing yourself to smile on a regular basis were proven to strengthen the immune system. Are you too hard on yourself? Try being your own loving parent, treating yourself as gently and with as much tenderness and consideration as you might treat your favorite child. Treat yourself to small, appropriate gifts when you've done something important for yourself, such as learning to test your own blood glucose or preparing a favorite meal using healthier ingredients. And think positively. If you are down in the dumps and thinking negative thoughts, try reversing those thoughts and considering the possibility that the opposite might be true. Take a deep breath, then turn that negative thought on its head for a moment.

Wrong: "Diabetes has ruined my life."
Right: "Diabetes has *not* ruined my life."

Wrong: "I'll never be able to control my blood sugar."
Right: "I *will* be able to control my blood sugar."

Wrong: "I won't ever be happy because I have diabetes."
Right: "I'll be able to live a *very* good life with diabetes."

This simple attitude adjustment is a trick that can affect your life in a positive way. Lighten up on yourself to relieve stress. Appreciate what you have. Although it's easier said than done, work to see the goblet of your life as being half full, rather than half empty. When something good happens to you, tell another person the news.

COUNSELING

Working with a good psychologist or religious counselor can benefit anyone who's under great emotional stress. Seek the services of a mental health professional when your problems are overwhelming your life. Identify your most pressing problems and concerns during counseling, and work to cope with them in a positive way. Professional counselors will listen carefully to you, and help you to sort out your personal issues. Talking with your rabbi, priest, or minister can be comforting too. Support groups can also be useful in dealing with the most emotionally stressful aspects of diabetes, which your medical team may not have the time to address.

Outside the ranks of professional counselors, don't forget to keep in touch with your friends, since they know you and care about you in a unique way. Many times, your friends may be able to see when you're under stress before you do because the effects of stress are often more visible to other people than to you. Ask your friends to tell you if you seem upset or under stress. Friends are important. Research shows that people who are not isolated from others generally live longer, happier, healthier lives.

PRAYER

It's not for everyone, but prayer can help relieve stress. Since the beginning of time, human beings have prayed for the health of themselves and their loved ones, turning to a higher power in an intimate, intuitive way. Praying is similar to meditation in its biochemical effects, according to author Herbert Benson, M.D., a Harvard University doctor who has written several books on meditation and healing. Dr. Benson argues that a belief in a higher power is a part of human nature, useful in countering our uniquely human ability to think about—and dread—our own mortality. As an example, Benson cites the so-called placebo effect, a false positive response that colors almost every medical experiment. The placebo effect occurs when research subjects receive no medicine or treatment, but show a positive response anyway. Dr. Benson calls this common response "remembered wellness," an example of the power of the mind and faith in medical treatment to bring about physical healing by itself.

Some proof exists that prayer has a direct connection with physical health. One ten-month study of the effects of prayer on two groups of heart patients at San Francisco General Hospital found that the group of patients that was prayed for by other people was much healthier, required fewer antibiotics, and was less likely to develop complications than the control group. A small, somewhat similar study of Type 1 diabetics at Healing Sciences Research International in Orinda, California, used a combination of therapeutic touch and prayer. Eleven out of sixteen Type 1 diabetics in the prayer and therapeutic touch group were able to reduce their insulin dosages, although the reductions were so small that they were not considered statistically significant.

Studies of churchgoers conducted over three decades showed that they have slightly lower blood pressure than do nonchurchgoers. Several studies have shown that people who are religiously committed also have lower rates of depression and anxiety-related illness.

WRITE IT DOWN

Writing down some of the stressful things you're experiencing can be very beneficial to your health. In a study conducted at Southern Methodist University, research studies have concluded that sharing feelings is good for the immune system. One group of students was asked to spend twenty minutes per day for four days writing about traumatic events in their lives. A second group was also asked to write, but instructed to focus on trivial events. The immune systems of the students who had disclosed their feelings were measurably stronger at the end of the four days. "Failure to confide traumatic events is stressful and associated with long-term health problems," wrote Dr. James Pennebaker, who headed the research team.

You can keep a diary anywhere, buying a lock-and-key model at a stationery store or keeping a secret file for yourself in your personal computer at home or at work. The benefits of writing down your feelings and thoughts may surprise you because they can lower stress.

SUCCESSFUL SELF-MANAGEMENT

According to Stanford University's Chronic Disease Self-Management Program, a person who successfully self-manages a chronic disease will:

- Set goals
- Make a list of alternative methods to reach the goal
- Make short-term plans or contracts to progress toward the goal
- Carry out the plans or contracts
- Check on progress weekly
- Make midcourse changes as necessary
- Use rewards when a job is well done

ALTERNATIVE TECHNIQUES

Some success at reducing stress has been experienced through alternative medicine techniques, such as the ancient Chinese techniques of *acupuncture* and *acupressure.* Acupuncture should be given by a person trained in its use because it involves taking the pulse in a special way and inserting needles into parts of the body. Acupressure is similar, but more easily applied at home. *Therapeutic touch,* a system of smoothing out the energy fields in the body, is popular with some nurses, but it does not involve much actual touching. *Massage* does involve touching by a massage therapist, and can relieve stress by reducing blood pressure and loosening up tense muscle groups, even if it does not directly lower blood sugar. *Pet therapy, music therapy, humor therapy,* and other alternative therapies are used to relieve stress among some groups of people who are chronically ill. No alternative therapy can cure diabetes, but some may relieve stress.

Since this list doesn't include every possible stress-relieving technique, don't lose sight of the things that have helped you relieve stress in the past. These can include activities that you simply enjoy doing, that are pleasant, and that are not physically harmful to you. Check with your medical doctor before you try anything new or unconventional, or if strenuous physical activity is involved. If you find something that works for you, share this information with your health-care team.

Self-management is an educational process that involves the use of five tools to help you control your diabetes. As later chapters will explain, these include blood sugar testing, lifestyle changes, and the use of certain medications. Relieving the high level of negative stress that accompanies diabetes is one important aspect of self-management. Exploring some of the techniques to relieve stress will give you a bit more control over your life. The next chapter deals with the most important single tool of diabetes management—blood glucose testing. Learning how to test and control your blood sugar will be quite important to you.

Chapter 6

TESTING

Blood Sugar Testing Is the
Most Important Thing You Can Do

~

BLOOD GLUCOSE TESTING IS THE SINGLE MOST IMPORTANT SELF-MANAGEMENT TOOL that you may ever have, because it allows you to know exactly what your blood sugar levels are at any one time. Using this knowledge, you may be able to spot problems and respond to them. This chapter explains the importance of keeping your blood glucose levels within a normal range, and spells out the symptoms and dangers of hypoglycemia and hyperglycemia. The basic mechanics of home glucose testing, the equipment that you will need, the frequency with which you should test, and some precautions to take are among the aspects of blood sugar testing included here.

One of the greatest breakthroughs in the management of diabetes in the past twenty years has been a method of blood sugar testing that is simple enough to be done at home and accurate enough to help the average person manage diabetes on a day-to-day basis. The first glucose testing meters appeared on the market around 1981. Although these first meters were expensive and cumbersome to use, like pocket calculators they have been simplified and improved in recent years. Right in your home, or in your office, thanks to great leaps forward in technology, you can obtain test results that are useful in controlling your blood sugar.

Since blood glucose levels far above or below normal are worrisome, glucose testing acts as a thermometer for people with diabetes. Blood sugar testing gives you an instant reading on your diabetes, much as a thermometer allows you to check a child's temperature to see if he or she has the flu. If your blood glucose is higher or lower than the level recommended by your doctor, testing lets you know that you need to bring it back within the normal range.

Every person's blood sugar levels fluctuate during the day. These fluctuations are somewhat predictable but they vary from person to person. Over a period of time, blood sugar testing allows you to see patterns of highs and lows that develop as your blood sugar levels rise and fall during the day. Understanding and controlling these fluctuations in blood sugar is called *pattern management,* which simply means recognizing your normal pattern of highs and lows, and developing a strategy to keep your blood sugars as close to normal as possible. When insulin is used, pattern management becomes more complicated because injections of insulin must be coordinated with meals and activities such as exercise, which also affect the blood sugar.

Although blood glucose testing only *measures* blood sugar, you can use these results in self-management. When you first test your blood sugars, you are like a new driver who begins to notice red or green stoplights on the road. Understanding these signals from your body will help you become a better driver.

GOOD CONTROL

It's important to recall that during the recent United Kingdom Prospective Diabetes Study, or UKPDS, people with Type 2 diabetes who maintained tight glucose control significantly reduced their risk of complications, achieving an 11 percent reduction in important HbA1c test levels, a 25 percent reduction in the risk of small blood vessel complications, and a 16 percent reduction in their risk of heart attacks. Tightly controlling blood pressure also resulted in a 24 percent reduction in complications. The Diabetes Control and Complications Trial in the United States, involving people with Type 1 diabetes, showed enormous benefits for tight control—76 percent less eye damage, 60 percent less nerve damage, and 35 to 56 percent less kidney damage. The mean average blood sugar for the group practicing tight control was 155 milligrams per deciliter, versus 231 milligrams per deciliter in the control group. The difference between these two numbers is quite significant. Clearly, good control of blood sugar will help you lessen your chances of long-term complications.

BLOOD SUGAR FLUCTUATIONS

Although the body requires some glucose in the bloodstream at all times, every person's blood sugars fluctuate a little during the day. In the average person without diabetes, blood sugar levels and insulin levels rise in lockstep to peak about an hour after eating. Blood sugar also rises slightly at night because the liver releases a bit of stored-up glucose into our bodies while we sleep. Most people with Type 2 diabetes have higher than normal levels of glucose because insulin isn't excreted and utilized by the body in the customary way.

Think of the average person's blood sugar as a truck pulling a trailer full of insulin. This truck-trailer combination goes up hills and down valleys several times a day, the linkage almost unnoticed because the blood sugar levels are so closely followed by and perfectly synchronized with the insulin.

For people with Type 2 diabetes, however, it's a different scenario. People with diabetes become extremely aware of the trailer full of insulin because theirs is not well synchronized or attached. At any moment, their insulin trailers may fly up too high, or skid to one side or the other, threatening to pull the truck off the road. Driving their truck-trailer rigs is a perilous proposition.

The great benefit of blood sugar testing is that it gives you the knowledge you need to synchronize your truck and your trailer. Self-management allows you to bring any perilous situation under control. With good self-management, you can learn to control blood sugar levels. This control will benefit your health.

NORMAL BLOOD SUGAR

In the United States, blood sugar levels are expressed in terms of *milligrams per deciliter,* abbreviated *mg/dl.* In countries such as Canada and Britain, where the metric system is more commonly used, these measurements are expressed in *millimoles per liter,* abbreviated *mmol/L.* To convert mg/dl to mmol/L, simply divide by 18. For instance, 100 mg/dl divided by 18 equals 5.5 mmol/L. In the United States, tests in your doctor's office and on your home blood glucose testing meter will express results in milligrams per deciliter. Laboratories and meters sold in other countries will express results in the measurements used in those countries.

The normal level of glucose in the blood is approximately 100 mg/dl, or 0.1 percent of the blood. This level fluctuates in all people. The normal range is 60 to 140 mg/dl, with increases after meals that drop as

BLOOD SUGAR

BLOOD SUGAR	FASTING	AFTER EATING
Normal range	>70 mg/dl (3.9 mmol/L)	<120 mg/dl (6.7 mmol/L)
Point of action	<60 mg/dl (3.3 mmol/L) or as advised	>140 mg/dl (7.8 mmol/L) or as advised
Call your doctor	As advised	As advised

glucose is absorbed. Over the course of a day, the average person's blood sugar levels will fluctuate a bit above and below the average, usually within a range of 30 to 40 mg/dl.

In the United States, the typical person without diabetes may have blood sugar readings in a range of 70 to 80 mg/dl before a meal, swinging up to 110 to 120 mg/dl about an hour after the meal, when the food breaks down into glucose and enters the bloodstream. Over two to three hours, the action of insulin helps lower blood sugar levels to approximately where they were before the meal. This pattern usually repeats at every meal. Since these are average blood glucose levels, a few points above average is of no particular concern. A variation of 10 points higher or lower than average is considered acceptable by most medical doctors.

In the person with Type 2 diabetes, however, blood sugar levels can soar many points higher than normal because the available insulin isn't synchronized with the blood sugar. In most people, blood sugar levels above 150 to 160 mg/dl (8.33 to 8.88 mmol/L) are often a serious concern because that's the point at which physical damage leading to complications is believed to begin. However, elderly people with diabetes may well have different glucose tolerance levels than do people who are younger because the human body changes with age. Fasting blood glucose levels increase by 1 to 2 mg/dl per decade after the age of thirty, and postprandial blood glucose levels can increase by 8 to 20 mg/dl per decade. At least one expert, Peter Porsham, M.D., a professor emeritus in medicine at the University of California at San Francisco, believes that damage from high blood sugar doesn't usually occur in elderly people unless glucose levels rise above 200 mg/dl (11.11 mmol/L). Other authorities argue that the role of high blood sugar in bringing on complications far outweighs the danger of low blood sugar, which increases the risk of falls and bone fractures in elderly people. No matter what your age, ask your doctor to set appropriate blood sugar level goals for you.

Many people can sense it when blood sugar levels are high. You may experience skin problems, feelings of fatigue, or tingling in parts of the body. A quick blood glucose test can confirm if high blood sugar is the cause of these feelings. With a few exceptions, blood sugar levels above 150 mg/dl (8.33 mmol/L) indicate a need for greater control.

Among the things that happen to your body when blood sugar is high, somewhere around 180 mg/dl (10 mmol/L), is that the kidneys begin to unload excess glucose into your urine, a process known as *glycosuria.* This is why diabetes is sometimes called sugar diabetes—the urine of a person whose blood sugar is elevated smells and tastes like sugar. *Diabetes mellitus,* the medical term for all types of diabetes, is a combination of *diabetes,* the Greek word for filter or siphon, and *mellitus,* the Latin word for sweet tasting. In the Middle Ages and for most of human history, the smell or taste of sugar in the urine was used to diagnose this disease.

Blood sugar levels can soar when you are sick, healing from surgery or an infection, or under extreme stress. Special precautions will be needed at these times. More about caring for yourself on sick days may be found in chapter 11.

Note that both short- and long-term risks are associated with off-kilter levels of blood sugar. The short-term risks are high or low blood sugar. The long-term risks are the many complications of diabetes. Avoiding these risks is why you must learn to check your own blood sugar levels, much like a good parent frequently checks her child's temperature when the child has a cold or the flu.

IMMEDIATE RISKS

The two immediate problems associated with blood sugar are unusually high and unusually low blood sugar. Although neither is fatal, both are quite serious. Unusually high or unusually low blood sugar is a call to action because either one will affect the brain, creating moments of memory loss, irritability, or depression. When you recognize your symptoms, you can take action to bring your blood sugar up or down.

Know *when* to call your doctor. *Always* ask the doctor who treats your diabetes to tell you at exactly what point you should consider your blood sugar levels to be dangerously high or dangerously low. Ask about the normal range for you, and for guidelines as to when you should call the doctor. Early on, write down exactly how many test results in a specified high or low range should make you immediately call your doctor.

The medical term for high blood sugar is *hyperglycemia*. With very high blood sugar, you may have a number of sensations that can warn you of the danger. The medical term for low blood sugar is *hypoglycemia*. With excessively low blood sugar, which is much rarer in people with Type 2 diabetes, you may feel it coming on or even faint in your tracks.

In this book, hyperglycemia is often referred to as high blood sugar and hypoglycemia as low blood sugar. The medical terms look and sound so much alike that it's easy to confuse the two, especially in the beginning, but everybody can understand high and low.

Down the river of self-management, high and low blood sugar are the two health hazards through which people with diabetes must steer their little boats. Learn what these hazards are, and how to recognize their symptoms in you. Share this information with your spouse or a trusted friend.

HIGH BLOOD SUGAR

High blood sugar is the greatest single danger for people with Type 2 diabetes because over time the presence of too much sugar in the blood is linked with long-term complications, such as heart disease, kidney failure, and blindness. Your power to raise and lower your own blood sugar is the greatest reason to check your blood sugar levels on a regular basis.

If you need another reason to control high blood sugar, note that you will continue to gain weight if blood sugars run high. The excess sugar in your blood will be stored in your body, some of it being converted into potentially dangerous fats called triglycerides. A feeling of depression may occur after several days of high blood sugar; this will affect the way you look at yourself and those around you, and probably hamper your efforts at self-management.

Unfortunately, many symptoms of high blood sugar are subtle and may easily be confused for something else, such as simply having a bad day at work or another minor health problem. This is why you should become attuned to your own body, and test your blood sugar. Learn to recognize the symptoms that you experience when your blood sugar is high.

One frequent symptom of high blood sugar is a stuffed, Thanksgiving afternoon feeling. Some feel a buzzing sensation in their bodies. Slow-healing cuts, sores, or infections can be warnings of high blood sugar. According to Richard Bernstein, M.D., author of *Diabetes Type 2, Including Dramatic New Approaches to the Treatment of Type 1 Diabetes,* other symptoms of high blood sugar *may* include confusion, headache, trembling hands, tingling in the fingers or tongue, buzzing in the ears, elevated pulse, unusual hunger, a tight feeling in the throat or near the tongue, clumsiness, less ability to detect sweetness in taste sensations, irritability, stubbornness, nastiness, pounding the hands on tables and walls, blurred vision, visual spots, double vision, visual hallucinations, visual impairments, lack of physical coordination, tiredness, weakness, sudden awakenings from sleep, shouting while asleep, rapid and shallow breathing, nervousness, light-headedness, faintness, feelings of unusual warmth, cold clammy skin, restlessness, insomnia, nightmares, paleness of complexion, nausea, slurring of speech, and a condition called *nystagmus* in which the eyes involuntarily jerk when sweeping from side to side. For some, blood sugar is elevated when the letters of the Arabic alphabet begin to look like they're written in Russian or Chinese. Other people walk into walls when their blood sugar is high. Some people become intensely angry and upset for no apparent reason. According to Dr. Bernstein, the symptoms of high blood sugar may occur in clusters or appear alone without other symptoms.

Since your symptoms will be unique to you, try to identify them with the use of home blood sugar tests. If it will help you remember, tell someone else or write down how you feel at the moment when your blood sugar tests unusually high for you. Ask your spouse or family members to tell you if they spot any symptoms of high blood sugar in you. Symptoms are distinctive to each individual—pay attention to your own body and learn to spot high blood sugar whenever you can.

If your blood sugar does become elevated, practice good self-management to reduce your stress, become more physically active, or adjust your eating patterns to bring it back under control. Medications can also help you accomplish this.

In the most rare and extreme instances of high blood sugar, such as when you have been ill over a long period of time, you may go into a *diabetic coma,* falling into unconsciousness for no apparent reason to those around you. In this case, you must be taken to a hospital emergency room for treatment.

Don't ignore high blood sugar. All the long-term complications of diabetes are believed to result from prolonged periods of high blood sugar or poor blood sugar control.

LOW BLOOD SUGAR

It's quite rare for people with Type 2 diabetes to experience low blood sugar reactions, which can include fainting at unfortunate moments, such as when you are driving a car. Repeated episodes of hypoglycemia can affect mental functioning. Low blood sugar occurs much more frequently in people with Type 1 diabetes, whose bodies don't produce any insulin.

Exceptions to this may include people with Type 2 diabetes who are taking hypoglycemic agents, and particularly those who are taking insulin. Striving for tight blood sugar control can increase episodes of low blood sugar. These people need to be aware of the possibility of low blood sugar, particularly when skipping a meal or during bouts of strenuous exercise that can rapidly lower blood sugar levels. You can raise blood sugar by eating a snack. However, if you faint and go into *insulin shock,* you'll need an injection of glucagon to snap you out of it, or medical attention in a hospital emergency room.

The possibility of low blood sugar reactions is one reason to take your diabetes medications as prescribed, and to never double up on doses if you miss one. If you're taking diabetes pills or insulin, skipping a meal can cause low blood sugar, which is another reason you should hew to your regular meal and snacking schedule as closely as possible. Timing of meals is particularly important if you are taking insulin.

Unusually long, strenuous bouts of exercise may cause blood sugar levels to fall quickly, which is why people who strenuously exercise should carry a snack with them when they work out. Drinking alcohol without eating and taking aspirin, barbiturates, and certain prescription drugs such as those that thin the blood can also lower blood sugar.

Symptoms of low blood sugar vary from person to person. They may include a feeling of being "out of sorts," sudden mood swings, loss of concentration, irritability, grumpiness, weakness, paleness, poor coordination, sweatiness, headache, or a feeling that something is wrong with the way that you're thinking. Some people experience no symptoms at all when their blood sugar levels drop.

TREATING LOW BLOOD SUGAR

If you test below 70 mg/dl (3.89 mmol/L) or whatever level your doctor has set, or you feel such symptoms of low blood sugar as confusion and shakiness, snacks can bring up your blood sugar quickly. Here are some recommended snacks:

- ½ cup apple juice or orange juice
- ½ cup carbonated soft drink (not sugarless)
- 1 small box of raisins
- 5 small sugar cubes
- 6–7 small pieces of hard candy (not sugarless)
- 3 glucose tablets or glucose gel
- 1 cup milk
- 1 tablespoon honey
- 1 tablespoon sugar

You can easily prepare for and prevent problems with low blood sugar. If you feel low blood sugar coming on, if you anticipate a sudden drop in your blood sugar, or if you test unusually low, just eat something sweet. Glucose tablets or gel, hard candy, raisins, and orange juice or fruit juice all work beautifully to lift and normalize blood sugar—see the chart above. The tablets and gel products have the advantage of being smaller and easier to carry, and you probably won't be tempted to snack on them.

If you have low blood sugar and don't respond to it right away, you may need the help of another person because untreated low blood sugar can make you confused, and may eventually cause you to lose consciousness. If this is even a possibility, such as when you are working out, let your exercise partner or trainer know how to recognize the signs of low blood sugar.

If you faint, that person should know that you need an injection of *glucagon,* a hormone that raises blood sugar. Glucagon comes in a kit containing a syringe and a special bottle of powdered glucagon; kits may be purchased with a doctor's prescription. It is not possible to overdose on glucagon. If low blood sugar is possible for you, you need to show family members or friends how to give you a shot of glucagon before anything happens, perhaps letting them practice by giving you an insulin injection. People who have never given a shot may not be able to do it in an emergency. If glucagon is not available when you pass out, ask another person in advance to call the paramedics and explain to them that you are diabetic and may have low blood sugar. No one should ever try to pour fruit juice or any liquid down your throat while you are unconscious.

Low blood sugar is rarely a concern for most people with Type 2 diabetes. But the off chance that this or another medical emergency may happen is reason enough to take precautions when you are traveling, such as wearing a medical ID bracelet and making sure your companions know that you have diabetes. Blood testing before you drive a car or fly a plane will alert you to any potential problems. Again, your spouse or significant other should understand how to help you in case of a medical emergency.

Good self-management and blood glucose testing will help you prevent excessively high or low blood sugar.

TESTING YOURSELF

To achieve good blood sugar control, you must periodically check your blood glucose levels to see how well you are doing. Your medical team will probably ask you to write down or record your test results, and will help you analyze them on a regular basis. Checking your blood glucose level periodically will give you and your doctor a sense of the fluctuating blood sugar rhythms of your body.

If your doctor asks you to keep written records of your test results, make an effort to keep them accurately. Some people are inclined to cook these numbers, using trickery or stretching the truth in an attempt to please their doctors, delude themselves, or avoid a lecture. Falsifying test results is not productive.

Although your home tests are important, note that the results you get may not be quite as accurate as the blood tests or laboratory tests given at your doctor's office. In some cases, test results may vary by as much as 20 percent. These variations are why you should take your home test results with a grain of salt, particularly the first reading that seems way too high or low. Simply repeat the test, and make sure your glucose meter meets all quality assurance criteria. Call the manufacturer's toll-free number if you have complaints or questions, or if you need help in checking your meter's accuracy.

Each regularly scheduled visit to the doctor who treats your diabetes should include a check of your blood glucose test results against the laboratory blood sugar results taken at the doctor's office. Remember to blood test yourself at the same time that the doctor's office does its test because if you don't, the comparison won't be accurate.

Portable blood glucose testing meters have been a boon to self-management. But don't be excessively hard on yourself over the results of home tests, which may be higher or lower than you expect. As a general rule, blood sugar levels of all people will be lower before eating

TESTING BLOOD SUGAR

Here are the basic steps to test blood sugar with the aid of a home glucose testing meter. The sequence and steps may vary according to the meter—use your meter as directed.

- Collect the materials you need, including blood glucose meter, lancet, strips, and record book.
- Wash your hands.
- Stick your finger to obtain a drop of blood.
- Start the timer running.
- Put the drop of blood on the strip and insert the strip into the meter as indicated.
- Read and record the results.

than after eating because the ingestion of food triggers a rise in glucose. Ask your medical doctor to recommend blood sugar goals for you. When practicing self-management, aim for the best you can do at the time rather than an impossible standard of perfection.

METERS

To test your blood sugar, you'll need a small inexpensive blood glucose testing meter, disposable lancets to prick your finger, and disposable blood testing strips for the machine to read. You may never enjoy pricking your finger, but you'll test like a trooper after a few tries.

Meters that can give you an accurate reading on your blood glucose without pricking your finger are in development, but not available yet. Some prototypes use laser beams to attempt to read blood sugar levels through the fingernail or wrist, or use other new technology to attempt a reading through skin patches. Another new meter tests on the forearm and other areas that have fewer nerves than the fingertips, resulting in less pain during testing. Perhaps the most advanced technology involves a continuous monitoring glucose sensor, approved in June 1999, which allows a sensor to be placed under the skin for as long as three days. This sensor is connected by a wire to the glucose meter, which can read glucose levels every few seconds and store them as frequently as every five minutes—producing hundreds of readings per day—perhaps the first step in continuous glucose control. Connecting the probe with an insulin pump itself could allow very tight control of blood sugar levels—even an alarm system that signals if glucose drops too low. No-stick glucose meters are expected to be very expensive when they first appear on the market, but prices will drop just as they did for today's testing meters. For instance, one new meter, recently approved for home use, uses a laser as a lancet and results in "nearly painless" tests, according to the manufacturer. First models will cost around $2,000.

Dozens of blood sugar testing meters are now on the market, including models sold by Johnson & Johnson, Bayer, Roche Diagnostics, Medisense, and Cascade. Check several before you buy. All newer models provide a digital readout. Most are battery operated and as small or smaller than a pack of playing cards. A few models even have the lancing device built into the meter. Several provide booklets in which to record your meter readings. A few come with a built-in memory that holds several dozen past readings, and some provide ways to enter information on insulin injections and exercise. Some meters can be connected to a personal computer through a special cable, allowing readings to be turned into easily read charts or graphs by using special software. A few meters have oversized, illuminated, or "talking" readouts, which are useful for elderly people or for people with limited vision. One meter gives verbal instructions for its use and can read the labels of certain insulin bottles aloud. Some can even be hooked up to a modem to send your test results to your doctor's office computer over the telephone lines prior to your appointment. Note that many home meters test and report glucose levels in whole blood, while tests at your doctor's office test blood plasma. Remember that whole blood readings are roughly 12 percent lower than plasma readings.

Your doctor normally won't advise you on which meter to buy. Your *diabetes educator* or *nurse educator* can tell you what's on the market or direct you to good sources of information. Some pharmacists, particularly those who have many customers with diabetes, may be able to explain the pros and cons of different models. Most mail-order houses specializing in diabetes supplies carry blood glucose testing meters.

Before you buy, consider how you will use your meter. Do you need to carry it to work or to meetings in your briefcase or handbag? Do you need it to help you remember your readings, which you may not have the time or inclination to record after every test? Do you like the color? When you consider the cost of the meter, lancets, and strips, which model can you afford? Check the costs that your health insurance will cover, and see if your selection of meters is limited in any way. The purchase of a meter and a portion of the daily supplies may be reimbursable. Medicare, for instance, will pay for a meter if you are taking insulin, and if your doctor gives you a written prescription for the meter as part of your treatment plan. More information on the financial aspects of diabetes can be found in chapter 14.

Most manufacturers are anxious to sell you one of their meters, just to guarantee a customer for their strips. The most you should pay for a meter is about $150. Many manufacturers offer some type of rebate; sometimes they'll even give you the meter for free. You'll purchase the blood test strips and lancets as needed, with the test strips usually supplied by the same company that manufactured your meter. The cost of the strips adds up—they're between 50¢ and $1 apiece. You use one strip each time you test, and more than one if you don't do it right the first time.

Lancets are short fine needles that should pierce the skin with minimal discomfort. They should be easy for you to hold and use. Some fit into a device that looks like a fountain pen, which pricks your skin with a spring-loaded snap. Since you're the only one using them, you may experiment with reusing lancets to save money, but remember that most get dull fairly quickly, and when they are dull the pricking is painful.

HOW TO TEST

You may be clumsy at first, but you'll get the hang of it. The basic procedure is to wash your hands, prick your finger with a lancet, place a droplet of blood on the test strip, test the strip, and read and record the results. Read and follow the instructions for testing that come in the package with your meter. Testing will take less time each day than brushing your teeth once you're comfortable with the procedure.

When you begin, you may unfortunately have to prick your finger more than once to get blood for the test. Don't be discouraged. You'll get better and faster as you go along.

To test, you'll need a good hanging droplet of blood. If you don't get a good drop, "milk" your finger by rubbing it down away from your hand with the fingers of your other hand and releasing it as you would the teat of a milk cow. If you can't get a good droplet from one location, try another. You may have to rub down your finger a few times to get a good droplet. Or you may be one of those fortunate people who bleeds easily.

Your choice of fingers to prick will depend upon your own manual dexterity and whether you're right-handed or left-handed. Make it as easy as possible on yourself. Pricking too far back on your finger might make it difficult to get the droplet of blood onto the test strip. Many people prefer to prick only the side of the finger, rather than the more sensitive fingerprint pad where you have more nerve endings. Techniques vary. Some people choose a couple of fingers that they use for testing each time. Some make several sticks into the same location because the callus that builds up also blunts the slight pain of injecting a lancet. If you do it this way, eventually the callus will stop you from getting the proper amount of blood, and you'll have to move on to another location and perhaps create another callus.

Selecting the right lancing device can be helpful. Some are less troublesome than others. Some will stick too deep, some not quite deep enough, because skin thickness varies from person to person. It's worth trying another type of lancing device if you have trouble with your first one—your diabetes educator or nurse may be helpful here. If you find a lancing device that's a bit more expensive but easier and more comfortable to use, it's probably worth the extra money to buy it.

Blood glucose meters usually work well for long periods of time. However, because they're mechanical devices, few work perfectly. Most manufacturers have a procedure for testing their meters' accuracy. They also have toll-free numbers to call if you experience problems with their products, and service people who can walk you through the testing procedure.

Remember that meter manufacturers want to keep their customers happy so that they can continue to sell them supplies. The majority will listen to your complaints or problems, and attempt to rectify them.

WHEN TO TEST

The doctor who treats your diabetes should recommend a blood glucose testing schedule for you, and ask to see your results during your regular visits. The more frequently you test your blood sugar, the more likely you are to achieve good control. But don't go overboard, either.

Testing your fasting blood sugar before you eat anything in the morning gives you a reading on your sugar levels without any food, but includes the small amount of glucose that your liver pumped out during the night, while you slept. Testing after meals tells you how the additional glucose generated by your meal is being assimilated. Blood sugar levels are often highest about an hour after you eat, when easily digested sugars and starches surge into your bloodstream and peak, before declining. If you test after eating and your blood sugars are lower than before you ate, your meter or your testing technique may be incorrect. If you use insulin before you eat, you could also experience a low reading.

The number of tests your doctor recommends may vary. In *A Touch of Diabetes,* authors Lois Jovanovic-Peterson, M.D., Charles Peterson, M.D., and Morton Stone recommend that people controlling Type 2 diabetes through diet and exercise alone test before breakfast and an hour after each meal every other day, or about three days a week. They recommend that people using diet, exercise, and diabetes pills test before breakfast and an hour after each meal every other day. For people using multiple insulin injections, they recommend testing before each meal and an hour after each meal every day.

Some doctors recommend that patients with Type 2 diabetes test a minimum of four times per day, one day a week. Others recommend two tests per day every day.

Testing before meals may be recommended by your physician if you're on medications such as diabetes pills or insulin because these tests can help tell you how well the medications are working. If you are taking diabetes pills or insulin, of course, you should also test your blood sugars any time you experience the recognizable symptoms of low blood sugar—feeling confused, sweaty, shaky, nervous, or weak. It will greatly help you to know the level at which you get these symptoms. If you really need to eat a snack, do so. The first rule of self-management is to take good care of your health.

Whatever your doctor's recommendations, your results may be kept in a record book, on forms provided by your health-care team, or in a file in your personal computer that you can print out and take to your doctor. If you've been testing as directed, an examination of your test results may yield clear, general patterns of high and low blood sugar, which may be modified through changes in eating patterns, stress reduction techniques, increased physical activity, or other means.

If your doctor doesn't recommend blood testing at home, ask why not. If your doctor says blood testing is not necessary, this physician

BLOOD GLUCOSE GOALS

Every person's blood sugar levels rise and fall during the day in response to the meals that they eat, their stress levels, and other factors. Your blood sugar levels will probably not be low when you first begin blood sugar testing, particularly if you are either young or elderly, in which case your blood sugar levels may be higher. Listed below are some good general blood glucose targets that people can aim for over the long term. However, always check with your medical doctor for blood sugar goals that are appropriate for you.

TIME	IDEAL RANGE	OKAY
Fasting	70–110 mg/dl (3.9–6.1 mmol/L)	60–120 mg/dl (3.3–6.6 mmol/L)
1 hour after a meal	90–150 mg/dl (5–8.3 mmol/L)	80–180 mg/dl (4.4–10 mmol/L)
2 hours after a meal	80–140 mg/dl (4.4–7.7 mmol/L)	70–150 mg/dl (3.9–8.3 mmol/L)
3 hours after a meal	60–110 mg/dl (3.3–6.1 mmol/L)	60–130 mg/dl (3.3–7.2 mmol/L)
Pregnancy—fasting	<90 mg/dl <5 mmol/L	
Pregnancy—2 hours after a meal	<120 mg/dl <6.7 mmol/L	

has not kept up with the times. Blood glucose testing has been an accepted part of good diabetes care for several years, for both Type 1 and Type 2 diabetes.

Remember that a glucose meter only reads blood sugar levels at the moment in which they are taken. As the Greek philosopher Heraclitis observed, you never step into the same river twice. Accept that your blood glucose levels rise and fall. Unless you're a fortune-teller, you won't be able to predict all your test results. Some blood glucose tests will be higher than you expect, some lower. Try to be philosophical. Don't fall into the trap of getting upset over tiny variations in test results. Try to look at these numbers as a scientist would look at raw data, rather than taking them as personal messages from the oracle about whether or not you're a "good diabetic." You're a good diabetic if you test, no matter what the results.

Remember, high blood sugar levels don't mean that you've suddenly become a bad person. Stress, certain foods, sickness, and many other factors can jack up blood sugar levels. If you get too upset over your own test results, you will further elevate your blood sugar. Look at blood sugar testing as a tool you can use to achieve control, rather than as a series of verdicts on whether you've been bad or good.

Every person's blood sugar levels are in constant flux, and each test that you administer reflects only that one moment in time. Always follow your doctor's recommendations on how many times to test, and when. Record the results as directed. Test your blood sugar more frequently when you are ill, and anytime you feel unusual.

LIFESTYLE ISSUES

Your doctor should recommend a glucose testing schedule that takes your work schedule and lifestyle into account. There should be some element of convenience in your testing schedule because you don't want to take on additional stress trying to test your blood sugar when you're pressed to do other things that are important to you, such as taking your children to school. Whether you're a farmer who spends long hours in the field on a combine during harvest season or a businessperson with a long commute to the office, you should test at times that fit comfortably into your schedule. Remember, too, that testing is a means of *preventing* low and high blood sugar. Testing yourself before you operate machinery is a good way of assuring your safety and that of others.

Since your body chemistry is unique, you may react differently to some foods than will other people, even other people with diabetes. You can track your own particular reactions to foods using blood sugar testing. Do you suspect that a four-cheese, pepperoni, and sausage pizza will unduly affect your blood sugar? Testing before and an hour after eating it will tell you how dramatically the pizza affected your blood sugar. When you learn something important about your blood sugar, share this information with your health-care team.

If you're exercising, especially strenuously, your doctor may advise you to test before your workout because aerobic exercise lowers blood sugar. Before you begin exercising, you may want to eat a light snack if your blood sugar tests low for you, around 80 mg/dl or whatever level your doctor or exercise physiologist has set for you. But try not to use the possibility of low blood sugar as an excuse to pig out.

As a general rule, aim for blood sugars as close to normal as possible because that's where the human body functions best. As directed by your doctor, you may be able to safely aim for blood glucose levels between 90 and 100 mg/dl (or 5 to 5.56 mmol/L) before eating, and 150 to 180 mg/dl (or 8.33 to 10 mmol/L) an hour or so after meals. Your medical doctor will help you set realistic goals for your tests.

Use common sense. If you test at 200 mg/dl (or 11.11 mmol/L) before lunch, don't eat a big, rich, carbohydrate-laden lunch. Take a short walk or do some exercise instead. Drink some water. Or you may modify your lunch to include only protein, such as a piece of chicken, and eliminate most of the carbohydrates (such as sugars and starches) to see if that helps bring your blood sugars back down.

This is a situation where it might help to know your reaction to particular foods.

Blood glucose testing is a self-management tool. Blood sugar levels will fluctuate. Your home test results can help you manage these fluctuations. Find a glucose meter that suits you, and test yourself as directed by your doctor and health-care team. You can use the results in many ways, such as for fine-tuning your eating style, which is the subject of the next chapter.

Chapter 7

FOOD

Changing Your Style of Eating Helps Control Diabetes

~

FOOD IS IMPORTANT IN MANY WAYS, PRIMARILY BECAUSE WHAT YOU EAT DIRECTLY affects your blood sugar levels. Controlling what you eat and when you eat helps your self-management, whether your goal is to lower weight or merely to control blood sugars. A registered dietitian or nutritional consultant, often an important member of your health-care team, may work with you to help you change your eating style in a way that suits your own life. The basics of nutrition and a few possible dietary strategies are examined here, as are tips to get you going and keep you going, and help get you through the hazardous holiday periods when temptation often appears.

We all need food to live, but food has both physical and psychological meanings for most people. Eating well, and in moderation, has long been recognized as important to good health. During the time of the Roman Empire, the poet Horace wrote in his *Satires,* "Now learn what and how great benefits a temperate diet will bring along with it. In the first place, you will enjoy good health."

ABOUT YOUR WEIGHT

In statistical terms, about 30 percent of all Americans are overweight. When people with Type 2 diabetes are considered as a group, a much greater proportion, more than 80 percent, are overweight. If you are within this group, your blood sugar levels may well return to normal if you can return to your normal or recommended weight. This is particularly true if you have had diabetes for less than ten years.

It's important to point out that blood sugar levels may drop *significantly* with even a small reduction in weight. Even if you are overweight, a loss of only 10 to 15 pounds will substantially lower your blood glucose levels. Almost instantly, you'll feel better with lower blood sugar. A decade or two from now, you'll have lowered your chances of serious complications. Adopt a more physically active lifestyle along with some reduction in body weight, and you'll feel better and reduce your risk of future complications even more.

Losing weight isn't an easy thing. Most obese people have been overweight for years. If you are overweight and have diabetes, you also have a metabolism that is out of kilter. Losing weight can be quite stressful, especially for older people. Overweight people almost always eat more of certain types of foods than they need to maintain a normal weight. Obesity can have a psychological dimension, too, which also must be considered if changes in eating patterns are to be maintained over time.

It's heartening to know that many people diagnosed with diabetes have been able to throw away their diabetes pills or insulin syringes simply by modifying their diets and becoming more physically active. True,

OPTIMUM WEIGHTS

Listed below are some optimum weight ranges for women and men, the U.S. government's *Dietary Guidelines for Americans*, released in 1995. Of course, women are typically shorter and have less body mass than do men. The lowest end of these ranges are appropriate for women with small physical frames; the upper limits are for men with larger, heavier frames. In the treatment of diabetes, your doctor or dietitian will help you determine a weight goal that is appropriate for you.

HEIGHT	WEIGHT IN POUNDS	HEIGHT	WEIGHT IN POUNDS
4' 10"	91–119	5' 9"	129–169
4' 11"	94–124	5' 10"	132–174
5' 0"	97–128	5' 11"	136–179
5' 1"	101–132	6' 0"	140–184
5' 2"	104–137	6' 1"	144–189
5' 3"	107–141	6' 2"	148–195
5' 4"	111–146	6' 3"	152–200
5' 5"	114–150	6' 4"	156–205
5' 6"	118–155	6' 5"	160–211
5' 7"	121–160	6' 6"	164–216
5' 8"	125–164		

you won't get a gold medal when you avoid wolfing down an extra-large piece of birthday cake. No one will hand you an Academy Award for taking a walk or an exercise class on a regular basis. But in the long run, changing your lifestyle to include a healthy, nutritious, well-balanced diet will increase the quality—and probably extend the length—of your life.

After all, thin people generally live longer. Actuarial tables prepared by insurance companies associate longevity with below-average weight. Amazing research studies conducted at UCLA and the University of Texas found that laboratory animals can extend their average lifespans by as much as 50 percent if they consume fewer calories. It's well established that people who are overweight have much higher rates of not only diabetes, but also heart disease, cancer, and other diseases. According to the U.S. Centers for Disease Control and Prevention, poor dietary habits and a lack of physical activity are associated with an estimated 300,000 deaths per year, ahead of every other known risk factor except the use of tobacco.

Nobody knows all the answers about obesity, which is epidemic in the United States. Sedentary lifestyles and high-fat, low-fiber diets are obvious suspects. Stress can be a factor. Genetics may be a factor in some cases. Research published twenty years ago in England found that people who are obese eat two to three times the amount of food eaten by lean people, and eat it two to three times as fast. This may be because overweight people don't allow themselves to enjoy the food they eat. As surprising as it may seem, many overweight people probably don't often give themselves permission to savor and enjoy their food.

Eating more food than your body can use is the root cause of being overweight. Reducing your intake of certain foods, increasing your intake of others, and adding more physical activity to your life will help you control your weight. Maintaining a healthy lifestyle produces great health benefits over time.

NUTRITIONAL SUPPORT

After you were diagnosed with diabetes, your medical doctor may have referred you to a *registered dietitian* or a *nutritionist* to help educate you about foods and help you plan meals. This is called nutrition therapy or diet therapy. According to a recent American Dietetic Association study, people with Type 2 diabetes saved an average of $1,994 apiece just from reduced expenditures for oral agents and insulin as a result of diet therapy. Helenbeth Reynolds, a registered dietitian affiliated with the University of Minnesota, says diet therapy often involves an average of two or three visits with a registered dietitian who should have laboratory test results from your doctor in hand. The first visit may be in a group setting to cover basic nutritional care and set goals. This is often followed by one or two individual sessions or follow-up visits to examine and individualize meal plans.

A registered dietitian or nutritionist may work with a particular doctor, have a professional affiliation with a clinic or hospital, or even have his own office. Your nutritionist should get to know you, and tailor his recommendations to you.

Since your body is unique and reacts in a distinctive way to food choices, you must use what you already know—and what you can still learn from a nutritional specialist—to choose the things you eat. Think of yourself as an athlete in training, advises Los Angeles dietitian Diane Woods, R.D. An athlete in training looks at food as an important aspect of achieving physical goals. If you plan nutritious meals for yourself and keep nutritious food in your home, you are on your way to a life of sensible, appropriate food choices that can help you control your blood sugar.

Even if you are not overweight, you may not be aware of all the food you eat, especially if your eating style involves snacks while watching television. For this reason, a registered dietitian or nutritionist may ask you to keep a written record of everything you eat for a few days. Once you know where you've been, planning your meals can take you where you'd like to go. You may change your eating style on your own, but consulting an expert may save you a lot of time and help you to succeed.

Your first appointment with a nutritional consultant should be set up by your doctor after you are diagnosed with diabetes. If your doctor does not recommend that you see a dietitian, act on your own. If you are in a health maintenance organization, ask your doctor to refer you to a dietitian even if he or she does not routinely do so. Remind your primary care physician that the American Diabetes Association recommends that you work with a knowledgeable registered dietitian experienced in treating people with diabetes, because nutritional therapy is integral to good diabetes care. Another way to locate a registered dietitian is to call the American Dietetic Association's toll-free telephone number, listed in Appendix A.

A registered dietitian might charge $75 to $125 per hour, with sessions ranging from half an hour to an hour. Medicare and Medicaid sometimes cover diet therapy if prescribed by a physician, but most health insurance companies approve diet therapy only on a case-by-case basis. An answer for a particular question might be found from services such as the American Dietetic Association's "Call an RD" service, which is a 900-number service that connects you by telephone with a registered dietitian at a cost of a dollar or two a minute.

Look for a dietitian who frequently works with people who have diabetes, and who understands current principles of nutrition. When you locate one, make an appointment for yourself.

THE ROLE OF A NUTRITIONIST/DIETITIAN

In a nutshell, you and your dietitian should go over your current food choices and figure out how to make them better. One meeting is not enough to do more than learn a few important principles. But learn what you can, work to apply it, and go back for follow-up appointments as recommended. Learn to use the telephone to ask for help with problems.

As a first step in this process, your dietitian or nutrition specialist may take a *diet history,* which will involve interviewing you about the foods you eat and writing down this information. You may also write a diet history yourself, as preparation for an interview with a diet professional or simply to make yourself more aware of your own eating patterns. If you're one of those people who can recall every meal and snack eaten for the past two weeks, then write down what you've eaten for the past few days and take it with you to your first appointment.

Another way of tracking your eating patterns is to keep a *food diary* of everything you eat for a period of time. You can estimate the quantities, but don't fudge on the details by leaving out a piece of candy here, or a bag of potato chips there. Be as honest and accurate as possible. A food diary is as good a place as any to begin thinking about the *quantity* of food you eat, and to start estimating the weight of some food items as you eat them. You may not be able to do this at every meal; for instance, if you're rushing to catch a commuter train after breakfast or having lunch with the ladies in your garden club on Wednesdays. But some meals *will* allow you time to begin your measuring. (See chart on p. 112.) As your self-management progresses, you may be asked to track several aspects of your care.

A food diary covering three days is a good way to begin examining your eating style. It may help to think of yourself as a detective, out to discover important clues that will solve the mystery of why you're overweight. If you don't already have a food scale, buy one and begin weighing those hamburgers and steaks. Take out your measuring cups, and begin measuring portions of fruits and vegetables. Count those slices of bread, count how many slabs of butter you spread on each slice, and so on. Yes, it's a lot of arithmetic. But counting and measuring even a few food items will give you a head start on *portion control,* which is necessary to control the amounts of food you eat. Portion control is a necessary skill, more easily learned than applied. Measure and write down quantities for awhile, until you begin to get the hang of it.

Looking closely at your eating patterns with the aid of a dietitian will give you an idea of what elements make up your eating style. Chances are, you can find ways to make it healthier and more nutritious.

Treatment Plan record for the week beginning Monday, _____ (date)

January 13th

Diet Log

Goal: 2,000 _____ calories/day

Date	breakfast	lunch	dinner	snacks	Exercise type/duration	Glucose Monitoring blood/urine time/result		Rx time	Notes
Mon.	1-ww bagel lt. creamch. 1/2 orange w/ nonfat yogurt	ham sand. on ww bread 1/2 c. chicken soup 1 apple 8 oz. 1% milk	4 oz. fl. steak green beans mushrooms 1/2 c. corn 1/2 cantaloupe	8 1/2 animal crackers-9:30 —— 1/2 banana	10 A.M. walk	8	190	√	cut on toe-called nurse-no problem
						5	172	√	
Tues.	1/2 c bran flakes 8 oz. 1% milk 1/2 banana	turkey sand. w/ mustard 1 oz. potato chips 1 1/4 c. melon	4 oz. baked chicken brown rice 1 c. carrots green salad	x —— 2 slices cake!!!	yoga class	8	177	√	Sorry-it's my husband's 50th birthday!
						5	194	√	
Wed.									

	breakfast	lunch	dinner	snacks	Exercise type/duration	Glucose Monitoring blood/urine time/result		R_x time	Notes
Thur.									
Fri.									
Sat.									
Sun.									

GOOD WRITTEN RECORDS

This self-care diary is designed to help you record information about your meals, snacks, exercise, home testing results, medications, and more.

Treatment Plan record for the week beginning Monday, _____ (date)

Date	Diet Log				Exercise	Glucose Monitoring		Rx	Notes
	Goal: _____ calories/day				type/duration	blood/urine	time/result	time	
	breakfast	lunch	dinner	snacks					
Mon.									
Tues.									
Wed.									

	breakfast	lunch	dinner	snacks	Exercise type/duration	Glucose Monitoring blood/urine time/result				R_x time	Notes
Thur.											
Fri.											
Sat.											
Sun.											

First and foremost, your dietitian should consider you. Tell this person something about yourself. Your work schedule, your regular commitments, even the types of foods normally eaten in your culture or by your ethnic group should be taken into account. Any medical problems or conditions that you have in addition to diabetes should be noted by your dietitian, as should any medications you take, including diabetes pills or insulin. All the major facets of your health and diet are important because the goal is to tailor a plan that you can maintain for your entire life. Also considered should be the types of foods you truly like, the types you dislike, as well as other factors, such as whether you're a vegetarian.

In your dreams, what do you wish to weigh? Do you wish to lose weight or maintain your current weight but lower your blood sugar? If you are overweight, it probably took you several years to gain the extra pounds. Plan to give yourself a fair amount of time to whittle down the excess. If your goal is simply to lower your blood sugar, develop a plan that will help you do that. Nearly everyone can substitute nutritious foods such as fresh fruits and vegetables for those foods that contain empty calories. And every person can drink more water, which is the beverage our bodies were built to drink.

Your relationship with your dietitian is important. In 1996, Denise Thomas, the chief dietitian at St. James Hospital in Portsmouth, England, wrote in *Practical Diabetes* that the success of many diets often turns on the relationship between dietitian and patient. Many times, she observed, the dietitian's recommendations will fail if they are not appropriate to that patient. Many diets fail because they are too restrictive or strict for the individual, causing the person to first break the diet, then feel guilty and eat even more.

As a rule of thumb, the more you know, the more you participate, the more you wisely choose appropriate foods for yourself, the greater benefit you will receive. Look at a change in eating style as a lifelong effort. You may choose to modify your diet following a few general guidelines, then fine-tune it later through something like an exchange group plan, which gives you a method of measuring and controlling the calories you eat.

Rest assured that changing what you eat is the safest method ever devised for controlling blood sugar. If you eat well and in moderation, a healthy eating style can even survive an occasional mistake.

As time goes by, you will learn through experience and blood sugar testing what foods raise your blood sugar. Avoid foods that jack up your blood sugar, or eat them only in very small amounts, as part of an otherwise healthy meal. Chinese food, pizza, and pretzels can send blood sugars soaring for some people, as can candies sweetened with sorbitol. A consistent rise in your blood sugar levels after eating a particular food indicates a strong blood sugar response to that food. If you suspect a particular food is a culprit, try cutting it out for awhile or substituting something healthier—for instance, thin-crust vegetarian pizza for deep-dish regular pizza—and see what effect that has on you. Foods affect us all differently. Even some people who eat the often-recommended bedtime snack of air-popped popcorn wake up with high blood sugar because most people need a combination of foods to slow down their glucose release.

If you have already begun blood sugar testing, you'll be happy to know that controlling your food intake for just a day or two might reduce your blood sugar levels and show up on home glucose tests. The results may be even better if you also adopt a more active lifestyle, especially one that involves a little aerobic exercise. You will do yourself and your family a big favor over time if you adopt a healthier, happier lifestyle.

THE JOY OF EATING

Eating and drinking are topics fraught with pleasure and pain for the human race. Eating food and drinking fluids are primitive, sensual, life-sustaining pleasures. For us, food has social and psychological importance. "You are what you eat," quipped the French gastronome Anthelme Brillat-Savarin, memorably expressing the undeniable bond between good food and a good life. But in our weight-conscious society, eating can also be a guilty pleasure since even a small weight gain can be humiliating, particularly for women.

We are prisoners of evolution. For thousands of generations, tribes of human beings spent much of their time hunting, gathering, storing, and preparing food, activities that involved the continuous use of the leg and arm muscles. Certain foods were not always available. To survive in this environment, the human body developed the ability to both maintain a fairly constant level of glucose and to store great quantities of fats, converted from the foods that were available. But in our sedentary culture, we have taken most of the physical labor out of gathering and preparing food. In industrialized societies, we can buy almost unlimited quantities of even those foods that our bodies require only in tiny amounts. In the animal kingdom, only human beings and domestic animals suffer from obesity.

On the most primal level, eating produces a feeling of comfort, filling the stomach and drawing blood from the brain and other parts of the body to help with digestion. Among the many chemical reactions that occur, food provokes the release of the neurotransmitter serotonin, which produces in the brain the sensation of being full. Since the production of serotonin slows down when you diet, mood changes and periods of carbohydrate craving can appear in people who have problems synthesizing this chemical. This chemically induced craving for carbohydrates is one reason why many people fail to stay on crash diets, which do not incorporate the beneficial changes in eating style necessary to stabilize weight over the long term.

Only a small percentage of people who try fad diets achieve long-term weight loss. Many people trying to lose weight can relate to a short, memorable couplet written by Samuel Hoffenstein, who may have set pen to paper in a moment of great gastric unhappiness:

> *"My soul is dark with stormy riot,*
> *Directly traceable to diet."*

The psychological aspects of dieting are quite complex, as are our society's attitudes about food.

MIXED MESSAGES

In this society, we give each other mixed messages about food. Women are expected to provide nourishing, comforting food to their families while remaining slim and beautiful as they presumably deny food to themselves. Men bring candy to their sweethearts, but are stricken with horror if their sweethearts gain weight. Your mother may have told you that sweets were "bad for you," yet your grandmother rewarded you with special holiday sweets, homemade cookies, or other carbohydrate-laden food surprises.

In many families, food becomes a reward, an inexpensive and tangible symbol of affection or love. Food becomes a bribe, a seduction, even a weapon. Too many of us reward (or punish) ourselves with sweet, succulent, forbidden food treats, even though the damage to the waistline is quite predictable over time. In the worst case, food can actually become an addiction, in which case self-help support groups such as Overeaters Anonymous or Weight Watchers may be of help.

Old rituals involving food are embedded in contemporary culture, where echoes of harvest festivals and successful hunts for game may still be seen. After a year of competitive sports, athletes traditionally have an awards banquet that involves a meaty feast as part of their reward. Religious and secular holidays, weddings, births, and deaths are often accompanied by huge banquets, with food a centerpiece of the event. Marketers of food and drink products capitalize on these old associations, producing glossy advertisements and television commercials that show trim, beautiful models rewarding themselves with beer, sweet soft drinks, and snack foods.

"I've been a diabetic for too long and cheated too often," confessed a woman who has been managing Type 2 diabetes for twenty years, and who now receives support and encouragement from her family. "My whole attitude now is just to ask myself, 'Is it worth it?'"

It's not easy to lose weight. In 1986, according to a consensus statement issued by the National Institutes of Health, only about 25 percent of people with diabetes who needed to lose weight were successful in losing 20 to 40 pounds. Only 5 percent were successful in losing more than 40 pounds. While strategies for changing eating patterns have changed and may be more effective, these statistics point out the difficulties involved in weight loss. Measured against these statistics, any weight loss is a victory. And keeping that weight off is a great success.

Some obesity may be genetic. Researchers at the Howard Hughes Medical Institute in New York examined a strain of overweight mice called *ob/ob* mice and found that they all carried a mutant *ob* gene, the first gene scientifically linked to obesity. Studies reported in the *New England Journal of Medicine* in 1995 theorized that some overweight people with diabetes may have a type of genetic flaw on the receptors of their fat cells, which causes them to burn calories more slowly than do normal people. This flaw, which research scientists believe may be due to a defective *Beta 3 receptor*, has been correlated with incidences of diabetes and obesity in studies of Pima Indians and with a study of obesity in Finland. Although these findings are preliminary and not definitively proven, they suggest that losing weight may be a lot more complicated than simply exercising a little willpower.

There's always more to learn when it comes to food. People who prepare their own food are more likely to succeed in changing their eating style than those who don't cook at all. The reason for this may be that cooks have more control over the ingredients that they use, as well as a direct physical connection with what they eat.

Remember that food is neither moral nor ethical. Hershey's Kisses are not intrinsically "bad" and carrot sticks not intrinsically "good." All items may be reduced to calories and therefore to numbers, says registered dietitian and diabetes educator Debbie Solomin, a diabetes nutrition specialist at Encino-Tarzana Hospital in Tarzana, California. Understanding and working with these numbers (expressed as calories) can help you change your eating style. Slow and steady permanent changes in eating style, rather than crash dieting, allow you to take weight off—and keep it off—over time.

DIFFERENT STROKES

Choose your own approach to changing your eating style because many approaches may work. The degree of sophistication that you put into fine-tuning your eating style is up to you.

The truth is, healthy eating is no longer much different for people with diabetes than for people without diabetes. In recent years, the U.S. Department of Health and most major health organizations such as the American Cancer Society and American Heart Association have all made recommendations for healthy eating. All of these organizations advise you to eat a variety of foods, particularly high-fiber foods such as fresh fruits and vegetables, and cut down on your consumption of fats, sugars, and salts. Alcoholic beverages are okay, they say, but always in moderation. And of course, most health organizations recommend that you maintain a desirable weight, which a healthy style of eating will help you achieve and maintain.

"Whoever was the father of a disease, an ill diet was the mother," observed the Elizabethan writer George Herbert, about four hundred years ago. Herbert could have been writing about diabetes because the link between this disease and diet is fundamental.

The American Diabetes Association and the American Dietetic Association have worked together to make recommendations regarding a good diet for people with diabetes. Some variation of these recommendations may help you achieve a balanced diet that includes a desirable mix of carbohydrates, fats, and proteins.

YOUR EATING STYLE

Many people already know what a healthy lifestyle entails. However, too many of us also blithely ignore what we know is in our best interest. Instead, we eat too many convenience foods, fast foods, greasy foods, rich foods, fattening foods, junk foods, and sweet and salty foods whose seductive flavors and convenience blind us to their nutritional shortcomings. Processing robs food of nutrients and often substitutes sugar, white flour, and fats in their place to provide flavor. One theory about why so many people are overweight in the United States is that people eat greater quantities of processed foods than they do unprocessed foods in an attempt to consume the vitamins, minerals, and other nutrients that are in such short supply in processed foods. And it's no secret that the typical American's eating style contains an unhealthy high percentage of fats, leading many men and women to become overweight.

Bad habits can be broken. An unhealthy eating style can be changed. Changing your style of eating is one of the challenges you may face in controlling diabetes. This is not a quick process. Even if your intentions are good, you won't wake up tomorrow morning looking as great as you did in high school. But you can improve. Think in terms of small steps, taken one at a time, rather than a single dramatic

WHAT AMERICA EATS

Type of Diet	Fat	Carbohydrates	Protein
Average American	40–50%	25–35%	25%
ADA Recommends	30% or less	50–60%	10–20%

leap into the evening gown or tuxedo that you wore years ago to the senior prom.

The way you approach this is up to you. Many people benefit from keeping written records during a period of weight loss because it helps them to see and track their progress. A study of people with Type 2 diabetes on weight-loss programs conducted at the University of Pittsburgh medical school showed that the people who kept meticulous written records lost an average of 37 pounds, while those who kept less meticulous records averaged a weight loss of only 10 pounds.

A healthy style of eating is not a magic pill or a quick fix, but over time it will make you a healthier person. A good eating style doesn't involve a tasteless diet of health foods. Instead, it should contain a nutritious balance of all types of foods, even, with moderation, the occasional savory sweet.

A healthy eating style for most people with diabetes is about the same as what is recommended for any person growing older, if that person wishes to avoid medical problems, such as high blood pressure and heart attacks. A good eating style combined with regular aerobic activity can actually slow down the physical degeneration that accompanies aging.

What *should* we eat? Almost always, the answer is a balanced diet. A balanced diet involves a good mix of foods, all of which contain nutrients such as carbohydrates, proteins, fats, plus all the vitamins, minerals, and other food elements that we need to remain alive. A quick look at the U.S. Department of Agriculture's Food Guide Pyramid, pictured on page 125, will help you understand the mix of foods that constitutes a balanced diet.

SERVING SIZES

The following examples demonstrate portion sizes of one serving of food in several categories of the USDA Food Guide Pyramid:

  2 to 3 ounces of cooked lean meat
  ½ cup of cooked dry beans
  1 cup of milk or yogurt
  1 ½ ounces of natural cheese
  2 ounces of processed cheese
  1 slice of bread
  1 ounce of ready-to-eat cereal
  ½ cup of cereal, rice, or pasta
  1 cup of raw leafy vegetables
  ½ cup of cooked or chopped
    vegetables
  ¾ cup of vegetable juice
  1 medium apple, banana, or orange
  ½ cup of chopped, cooked, or canned fruit
  ¾ cup of fruit juice

The Food Guide Pyramid is designed to give you an easy-to-understand guide to healthy eating. It explains simply the *types* and *quantities* of food choices that contribute to a healthy diet. Note that grains, fresh fruits, and vegetables are at the wide base of the pyramid—the message is that we should consume many more servings of plant products than we do of all other types of foods. Dairy products, eggs, and meats are needed in lesser quantities. Fats, including

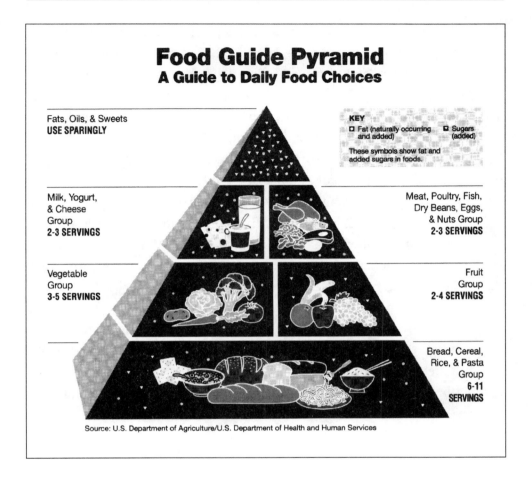

Food Guide Pyramid
A Guide to Daily Food Choices

**Fats, Oils, & Sweets
USE SPARINGLY**

KEY
□ Fat (naturally occurring and added)   ☑ Sugars (added)

These symbols show fat and added sugars in foods.

**Milk, Yogurt, & Cheese Group
2-3 SERVINGS**

**Meat, Poultry, Fish, Dry Beans, Eggs, & Nuts Group
2-3 SERVINGS**

**Vegetable Group
3-5 SERVINGS**

**Fruit Group
2-4 SERVINGS**

**Bread, Cereal, Rice, & Pasta Group
6-11 SERVINGS**

Source: U.S. Department of Agriculture/U.S. Department of Health and Human Services

vegetable oils, butter, margarine, and lard, top the pyramid because we need only tiny quantities of these to maintain a balanced diet. Try to think of yourself as a vegetarian who occasionally eats animal products. Thinking of meat, chicken, or fish as a side dish rather than a main course will help.

To better understand this concept, glance at the Food Guide Pyramid suggestions for the *quantity* of foods to eat. If you can change the mix of foods that you eat to approximate these recommendations, you'll be taking a step toward a balanced diet—and better health.

Every day, if you eat 6 to 11 servings of the bread, pasta, cereal, and rice group; 3 to 5 servings of vegetables; 3 to 4 servings of fruits; and so on, you will be eating a well-balanced diet. Note that the serving sizes are small—one slice of bread; 1 ounce of cereal; half a bagel; half a cup of pasta or rice; half a cup of cooked fruits or vegetables; a medium-sized apple or banana; 2 to 3 ounces of lean meat, chicken, or fish; a cup of milk; 2 ounces of low-fat cheese; and modest amounts of butter, alcohol, high-fat salty snacks, or candy.

The Food Guide Pyramid isn't a complete answer as much as it is a great place to begin. The approach is that some food choices are superior to others. Nonfat or low-fat dairy products are much lower in fat than are other dairy products. Choosing your protein from dried beans, tofu, fish, or chicken is generally better than choosing eggs or marbled red meat, which contain more cholesterol and fat. Most people with diabetes should cut way back on highly concentrated, quickly absorbed sweets, including all types of sugar, molasses, and the syrups in canned fruits. Unprocessed foods are better choices than highly processed foods. Other distinctions and choices, such as between the different types of fats and oils, are also helpful in designing a plan of healthy eating.

FOOD FACTS

Human life can be sustained on a mixed diet containing many types of plant or animal foods. In fact, the body *requires* a mix of food items to survive, ideally a balanced diet. The three basic *macronutrients* are carbohydrates, proteins, and fats. Many foods contain all three.

All three macronutrients work differently in the body. Some of each is essential for good health. All macronutrients contain *calories,* which are units of potential food or heat energy. A calorie is the amount of energy needed to raise the temperature of 1 kilogram of water 1 degree centigrade. Since people have different energy requirements depending on their age, gender, weight, activity level, and lifestyle, most diets are expressed in terms of calories consumed per day, as in 1,200 calories per day, 1,600 calories per day, or 2,000 calories per day.

For the person with diabetes, the most important thing to understand is that all three macronutrients convert at least partially into glucose. But carbohydrates, proteins, and fats convert into glucose in different proportions and at different rates of speed. Excess quantities of carbohydrates, proteins, or fats are stored as various types of fats, or triglycerides, in the body.

Facts About Macronutrients

Nutrient	Calories/Gram	% to Glucose	Maximum Glucose
Carbohydrates	4	100	1–1.5 hours
Protein	4	60	2–2.5 hours
Fat	9	10	5–6 hours

Carbohydrates, proteins, and fats all serve slightly different functions in the body.

CARBOHYDRATES

Carbohydrates are used for quick energy. Sugars are the simplest form. Starches, or complex carbohydrates, are carbohydrates that are more chemically complex. Although complex carbohydrates are often more nutritious than are simple sugars, in 1994 researchers established that both convert to blood sugar at about the same rate, the opposite of what was assumed to be true for many years. What this means is that even very sugary foods such as soft drinks, which have few nutrients or vitamins, convert to glucose at about the same rate as a vitamin-rich fruit like an apple or an orange. Since carbohydrates are smaller molecules than proteins or fats, they are more easily absorbed into the bloodstream, where their glucose reaches its high point between an hour and an hour and a half after eating. Sugars include sucrose, as in white table sugar; fructose, or fruit sugar; lactose, or milk sugar; maltose, or beer sugar; and the sweetener dextrose. (The average American eats about 20 teaspoons of sugar per day, the equivalent of 320 nonnutritional calories, but many people don't realize the quantity of sugar they consume because it's added to processed foods.) Starches, or complex carbohydrates, include potatoes, corn, peas, pasta, rice, bread products, and legumes. Carbohydrate consumption is recommended at 50 to 60 percent of total food intake, which is higher than the typical American diet. Of this, recommendations suggest a maximum of 10 percent of the total food intake be in the form of sugar.

PROTEINS

Proteins, sometimes called the building blocks of life, are needed for the growth of cells such as hair and hormones, in many organs of the body, and in a number of complicated chemical processes such as the repair of cells. The metabolism slows with age, reducing the need for protein. The American Diabetes Association recommends that people with diabetes limit their protein intake to 10 to 20 percent of the total diet, lower than the typical American diet. Animal products such as chicken, fish, meat, milk, and eggs contain protein, as do some plant foods such as grains, rice, and legumes. Proteins convert more slowly into glucose than do carbohydrates, reaching their high point between two and two and a half hours after a meal.

FATS

Fats are the most concentrated source of calories, which is why most diets advise people to cut the amount of fats that they eat. Too many fats make you fat. However, fat supplies the essential fatty acids used in the body to insulate us against heat and cold, and to carry fat-soluble vitamins such as Vitamins A, D, E, and K. Saturated fats are the type of fat that should be controlled or reduced in the diet for maximum health. The American Diabetes Association recommends that people with diabetes eat a maximum of 30 percent of their total calories in the form of fats, less than the typical American diet. In addition, the ADA recommends that at least two-thirds of these fats be in the less harmful monounsaturated or polyunsaturated form, which includes olive oil, canola oil, and corn oil. This recommendation leaves less than 10 percent of total calorie intake in the form of more harmful saturated fats, usually solid at room temperature, such as lard, butter, and tropical oils such as palm oil. If your cholesterol or triglyceride levels are elevated, the ADA recommends that only 20 percent of total calories be from fats. Although fats are concentrated calories that contribute greatly to weight gain, the good news is that only a small percentage of fats converts to blood sugar. Glucose from fats peaks very slowly, five to six hours after eating, and then slowly disappears from the bloodstream.

Learning which foods contain calories in the form of carbohydrates, proteins, and fats, and planning meals to create a balanced diet is the great leap forward in making any fundamental change in eating style.

YOUR PLAN

Medical doctors and dietitians are nowhere close to agreement on the proportions of carbohydrates, proteins, and fats that should appear in the diets of people with diabetes. This is probably as it should be, since each person's body is different; any changes you make in your diet should be appropriate for you. If you wish a copy of the American Diabetes Association's latest recommendations, call its toll-free number, listed in the "Other Resources" appendix at the back of this book.

As a general rule, people who need to lose weight will need to develop a diet that gives them a few less calories to eat than they burn off each day. If you can cut 250 to 500 calories per day from your diet by lowering portion sizes, particularly of the most fattening items, some of your weight will disappear. Participating in a weight-loss diet that you've helped design, especially one that aims at a slow reduction in weight, should result in significant weight loss over time, particularly when combined with a more physically active lifestyle.

One way to choose items that are low in calories and fats is to read food labels. For instance, comparing the standardized labels that must appear on the backs of milk cartons (and other food items) will show you that regular milk gets 30 percent of its calories from fat, while low-fat 2% milk gets 20 percent, 1% milk gets 10 percent, and nonfat milk gets negligible calories from fat.

Most dietitians recommend three meals plus snacks at regular intervals during the day for all people with diabetes. This is because spreading out your meals and snacks helps even out fluctuations in blood sugar. For the same reason, do not miss a meal. Skipping breakfast is associated with being overweight. It may surprise you to learn that people who always eat breakfast tend to be thinner than average.

A CHOICE OF PLANS

Exchange lists, food points, constant carbohydrates, and fat and carbohydrate counting are the approaches most commonly used by dietitians in menu planning. All of these approaches work for some people. One may suit you. All require time, thought, and effort to learn and implement. All involve planning, being aware of the differences among foods, selecting food items, and measuring portions. Even good cooks don't think naturally in terms of individual portions of food. Could you identify a 3-ounce steak on the meat rack in your supermarket, or place 1 cup of green beans onto your plate? Measurements such as these are important in diet plans. A greater awareness of the weight and volume of various portion sizes comes from simply reading the backs of food packages to size up the portions inside. The most accurate method is to use a scale and cups to measure what you eat.

In order to control what you eat, you need to know the servings or portions of various foods and their caloric values. If you aim for a particular number of calories each day, a knowledge of serving portions and the caloric values of foods gives you all the information you need to plan your meals in advance. As you plan ahead, you need to add these numbers up until they reach 1,600 calories per day or whatever goal you have developed with your dietitian or nutritionist. Then you need the discipline to shop correctly and stick with the plan.

All dietary approaches restrict total calories. Whether the aim is to lower blood sugar or to eventually reduce your weight, any basic change in eating style should strive to provide all the nutrients you need for good health.

SYSTEMS TO USE

The exchange list system is the one system recommended by both the American Diabetes Association and the American Dietetic Association. This strategy involves planning servings based on lists of foods that have approximately equal calorie, carbohydrate, and fat content. Exchange lists allow a variety of food choices each day, and provide the option of substituting foods for others of equal exchange point value. The idea is that you can exchange a serving of complex carbohydrate for a serving of a sugar or a fruit at the same meal because they're of equal value in the exchange list tables and have a similar effect on blood sugar. The exchange list system is flexible, which has more appeal to most people than following a rigid meal plan every day.

Milk, vegetable, fruit, bread/starch, meat, and fat exchange categories are included in the exchange lists, with exchanges limited to foods of approximately the same caloric value. Books explaining the exchange list system are available from your dietitian, doctor, or diabetes educator, or from the American Diabetes Association or the American Dietetic Association. Exchange list literature explains the portion sizes of various foods, another key to making the exchange list system work. Exchange lists are available for ethnic foods and fast foods, and come in English or Spanish versions. The original Weight Watchers program is similar to the exchange list plan.

Another option, the constant carbohydrate strategy, involves setting a goal of so many servings and grams of carbohydrates per day, and counting the grams of carbohydrates in each food item. This system has become more popular since the American Diabetes Association changed its eating guidelines in 1994 to allow for the fact that sugars and starches affect the blood sugar in approximately the same way.

Fat gram and carbohydrate counting methods do a similar thing with fats and carbohydrates. Fat gram counting aims to reduce the intake of fats at each meal to certain levels. Fat gram counters are used to show you how many grams of fat are contained in various foods. Cutting the grams of fat you eat each day will help you to lose weight, which helps you utilize your available insulin. Recent research has shown that for some individuals, cutting down their total fat intake is more important than cutting calories when the goal is to lose weight.

The food points system assigns points to various foods, using the equivalent of 75 calories for 1 food point. This makes 22 calorie points the rough equivalent of 1,600 calories per day and 40 calorie points roughly equal to 3,000 calories per day.

It can't be overemphasized that *all* weight-loss programs work best when done in tandem with a program of daily physical activity or exercise, which also helps reduce blood sugar levels.

Always use moderation and common sense on your diet.

GLYCEMIC INDEX

Although it doesn't relate directly to weight loss, the glycemic index does relate to blood sugar. Actually, there are several glycemic indexes. All seek to quantify the rate at which various foods convert to glucose and enter the bloodstream.

In 1981, David J.A. Jenkins, D.M., and his associates at the University of Toronto in Canada published the first Carbohydrate Glycemic Index, measuring how quickly sixty-two different foods raised blood sugar. Under the Jenkins system, 100 is the top figure, assigned to glucose. Beans and dairy products are generally low on the glycemic index, but interesting variations occur within food categories. Among the grain products to which Jenkins assigned an index value, for instance, whole wheat pasta is 42, white pasta 50, brown rice 66, white bread 69, whole wheat bread 72, and white rice 72.

In a more recent glycemic index, which uses white bread as the standard of 100, one of the lowest index values is given to *chana dal,* an Indian food similar to chickpeas, which gets a 12 on the glycemic index. *Nopal,* the prickly pear cactus, gets a 10, and is the lowest known food on a glycemic index.

Unfortunately, all glycemic indexes have flaws. Because each person's body chemistry is different, we all convert foods into glucose at our own pace. But the glycemic index can be a good way to start thinking about the effects of various foods on blood sugar.

THE GLYCEMIC INDEX AT A GLANCE

This glycemic index developed at the University of Toronto measures the rate at which various foods convert to glucose, which is assigned a value of 100. Higher numbers indicate a more rapid absorption of glucose. This is not an index of food energy values or calories.

SUGARS

Glucose	100
Honey	87
Table sugar	59
Fructose	20

SNACKS

Mars bars	68
Potato chips	51
Sponge cake	46
Fish sticks	38
Tomato soup	38
Sausages	28
Peanuts	13

CEREALS

Cornflakes	80
Shredded wheat	67
Muesli	66
All bran	51
Oatmeal	49

DAIRY PRODUCTS

Ice cream	36
Yogurt	36
Milk	34
Skim milk	32

ROOT VEGETABLES

Parsnips	97
Carrots	92
Instant mashed potatoes	80
New boiled potato	70
Beets	64
Yam	51
Sweet potato	48

PASTA & RICE

White rice	72
Brown rice	66
Spaghetti (white)	50
Spaghetti (whole meal)	42

BREADS		LEGUMES	
Whole wheat	72	Frozen peas	51
White	69	Baked beans	40
Buckwheat	51	Chickpeas	36
		Lima beans	36
FRUITS		Butter beans	36
Raisins	64	Black-eyed peas	33
Banana	62	Green beans	31
Orange juice	46	Kidney beans	29
Orange	40	Lentils	29
Apple	39	Dried soybeans	15

CARBOHYDRATE RESTRICTING DIETS

Some good doctors still recommend the use of unusually low-carbohydrate diets, which were used to treat diabetes during Victorian times. Some of these utilize quick severe carbohydrate restrictions as a first step in changing the eating style, a strategy designed to quickly bring blood sugars under control. A few use medically supervised low-carbohydrate diets as a long-term strategy for weight loss.

Doctors and dietitians at the Presbyterian Diabetes Center in Albuquerque, New Mexico, sometimes recommend the Fast Fast to bring blood sugars under control. Not a complete food fast, the Fast Fast is actually a fast from sugars and starches for three to five days. It's given under a doctor's supervision, and requires testing blood sugars at least twice a day. Type 2 diabetics undergoing a Fast Fast eat a small serving of meat each day, plus all the salad with low-fat dressing and sugar-free gelatin that they want, as well as unlimited sugar-free soda, coffee, and tea. The Fast Fast requires the person to drink at least eight large glasses of water per day, according to nurse educator Virginia Valentine, coauthor of the book *Diabetes Type 2 & What to Do,* along with June Biermann and Barbara Toohey. After a few days, people coming off a Fast Fast begin adding low-carbohydrate vegetables such as broccoli, green beans, and so on, one at a time, while testing and observing each food's effects on the blood sugar. People taking diabetes pills or insulin who do the Fast Fast need special attention and coaching from their health-care teams.

Yehuda Handelsman, M.D., a diabetologist and an instructor at the University of Southern California, recommends that his new patients fast from food for twenty-four hours, then go on a high-protein diet for a week or two to bring their blood sugars under control. After that, his patients add carbohydrates and fats. Among other things, Handelsman says that protein induces the production of insulin, a reason why every meal eaten by a person with diabetes should contain a bit of protein. After achieving blood sugar control, Handelsman recommends a diet of 25 to 30 percent protein, 40 to 45 percent carbohydrate, and 35 to 40 percent fat. Monounsaturated fats such as those found in olive oil, canola oil, and walnuts are preferred. Handelsman cites a research study published in *The New England Journal of Medicine* in which eleven patients substituted olive oil for carbohydrates and experienced a significant improvement in blood sugars. Garlic is another good food to include in the diet, he adds, because some tests show it can reduce cholesterol levels 8 percent by reducing cholesterol production in the liver.

Los Angeles endocrinologist Calvin Ezrin, M.D., recommends a diet that strictly limits carbohydrates over the long term, producing some remarkable losses of weight when undertaken under a doctor's supervision. According to Ezrin, severely limiting carbohydrates forces the body to burn fats, the body's preferred fuel. The Ezrin diet involves a very low intake of 20 to 35 grams of carbohydrates per day for the first two weeks, increased in increments after that. Ezrin's diet does throw the body into a state of "beneficial" ketosis, causing ketones produced by the utilization of fat to be excreted in the urine. However, Ezrin says that this mild ketosis is not medically dangerous when the diet is supervised. People following the Ezrin diet take vitamin and mineral supplements, including vitamins C and B complex as well as calcium and salt. Dieters are advised to exercise to their natural limits, drink lots of water, and take other precautions as recommended by the doctors supervising their weight loss. The Ezrin plan is spelled out in *The Type 2 Diabetes Diet Book,* cowritten with health writer Robert Kowalski.

VEGETARIAN DIETS

Vegetarian diets can be extremely beneficial when properly supervised because fruits and vegetables contain almost all the vitamins you need, plenty of fiber, and no saturated fat or cholesterol. Vegetarian diets can help control heart disease and may help people lose or control their weight.

Although our stomachs can handle both plant and animal products, some anthropologists believe that humans are primarily plant eaters because the human intestinal tract is much longer than that of animals who primarily eat meat. A longer digestive tract has evolved, this theory goes, because of the greater amount of time that it takes to digest and pass plant foods, which contain fiber. Short digestive tracts are more often found in meat-eating animals because the digestion of meat produces toxins that need to be quickly expelled from the body for the organism to survive. In addition, human teeth resemble the teeth of animals who primarily eat plants, a difference you'll notice by comparing your teeth with those of carnivores, such as cats and dogs, and plant-eating animals such as horses and cows. And from an ecological point of view, because the supply of land is limited, it's much more efficient for farmers to grow edible plants than to grow plants to fatten up farm animals. You can grow 10 tons of potatoes on an acre of land, for instance, but the same acre can only produce 165 pounds of beef.

Special precautions must be taken by vegetarians, who must make a concentrated effort to replace nutrients such as the calcium they might get from dairy products, or the iron and protein they might get from meats, even though vegetarians may require less of these vitamins, minerals, and nutrients than do people who eat animal products. Vitamin B-12 levels sometimes drop in vegetarians, making B-12 shots or supplements necessary. No single plant food has the nutritionally complete protein found in animal products, although many common food combinations, such as rice and beans, do equal a complete protein. For these reasons, the guidance of a registered dietitian or nutritionist is recommended for anyone beginning a *vegan* diet, in which no animal products are eaten. *Lacto-vegetarians* have an easier time eating a balanced diet because they allow themselves to eat dairy products. *Lacto-ovo-vegetarians* eat dairy products as well as eggs.

In 1986, the American Dietetic Association released guidelines for a vegetarian diet that included the following remarks:

> A considerable body of scientific data suggests positive relationships between vegetarian lifestyles and risk reduction for several chronic degenerative diseases and conditions, such as obesity, coronary artery disease, hypertension, diabetes mellitus, colon cancer, and others. . . . Vegetarians also have lower rates of osteoporosis, lung cancer, breast cancer, kidney stones, gallstones, and diverticular disease.
>
> Although vegetarian diets usually meet or exceed requirements for protein, they typically provide less protein than non-

vegetarian diets. This lower protein intake may be beneficial, however, and may be associated with lower risk of osteoporosis in vegetarians and improved kidney function in individuals with prior kidney damage. Further, a lower protein intake generally translates into a lower fat diet, with its inherent advantages, since foods high in protein are frequently also high in fat.

It is the position of the American Dietetic Association that vegetarian diets are healthful and nutritionally adequate when appropriately planned.

James Anderson, M.D., a physician from Lexington, Kentucky, has developed an alternative. Dr. Anderson, an early believer in oat bran, now champions high-fiber diets, especially for overweight people who have Type 2 diabetes. His high-carbohydrate and fiber nutrition plan features very low-fat meals; he says that if the diet is followed it will help lower weight, blood sugar, and cholesterol. Anderson recommends that people with diabetes eat up to 70 grams of fiber per day, more than four times the average American's consumption of 10 to 15 grams of fiber per day. He believes improved glucose control and lower cholesterol levels result from a greater consumption of foods containing soluble fiber such as oat bran, beans, peas, potatoes with skin, brussels sprouts, corn, zucchini, prunes, apricots, bananas, blackberries, and barley. Anderson observes that replacing 6 ounces of meat with 1 1/2 cups of beans will reduce total calories by 200, reduce dietary fat by 10 percent, and add 10 to 15 grams of fiber. This is explained in his book *Diabetes: A Practical New Guide to Healthy Living*.

The well-publicized program that Dean Ornish, M.D., developed in San Francisco for reducing heart disease involves a diet that is basically vegetarian, with a few exceptions such as fish and yogurt. Ornish's program is said to reduce deposits of plaque in the blood vessels, partially

ADDING MORE FIBER TO YOUR DIET

Fiber may help you lose weight because it produces that satisfied feeling of being full. Fiber helps move food through your body, and may prevent other diseases. Here are a few simple ways to add fiber to your diet:

- Eat more fresh fruits and vegetables—at least five servings per day are now recommended by major health organizations.
- Cook vegetables and fruits such as potatoes and apples with their skins on whenever possible, and eat the skins.
- Choose whole grain bread and whole grain cereals instead of food products made with refined flour.
- Add a spoonful of unprocessed bran, wheat germ, or oat bran to food items such as salads and hot cereals.
- Drink more water because water helps you to use the fiber more effectively.

by permitting only 10 percent of total calories to be drawn from fats, with almost all of those in the unsaturated form. This diet is far too restrictive for some people. However, in addition to diet, Ornish employs a multidisciplinary approach to heart disease that involves the use of yoga, meditation, communication training, and other stress-reduction techniques that can work together to reduce heart disease without surgery or drugs.

ABOUT FIBER

Whether or not you think of yourself as a vegetarian, fiber is important for good health. Increasing your consumption of fiber is recommended by the American Heart Association and the American Cancer Association because high-fiber, low-fat diets help prevent heart disease and cancer. Since heart and vascular problems are among the most deadly complications of diabetes, this is reason enough to include plenty of fiber in what you eat. Although 25 to 30 grams per day are recommended for most people, even this amount of fiber can cause intestinal discomfort and bothersome flatulence in some people.

Unfortunately, small increases in fiber consumption won't make much difference in your blood sugar. The current consensus is that although certain types of soluble fiber may delay the absorption of glucose, fiber in itself doesn't have much effect on blood sugar. Fiber does have the great benefit of making you feel full, so increasing your fiber intake may help you lose weight. Since fiber is found in healthy foods such as grains, fruits, and vegetables, adding fiber may help you change your eating style from a hodgepodge of junk food and empty calories to healthier balanced meals that make you feel like you've eaten something. Eating more foods that contain fiber may benefit people with diabetes in more subtle ways. A 1990 study published in *The American Journal of Clinical Nutrition* showed that a high-carbohydrate, high-fiber diet increased insulin sensitivity and lowered cholesterol.

When it comes to how you feel after eating, a calorie is not necessarily just a calorie. A study published in the prestigious British medical journal *The Lancet* measured the effects of meals of apple juice, applesauce, and apples on patients at the Royal Infirmary in Bristol, England. Each apple dish contained identical calories. Subjects ate the food and were tested. Blood sugar levels rose about the same for each form of apple, but fell or rebounded quickly after the juice, with less rebound for the applesauce and none at all for the patients who ate the apples. Respondents reported that apples were most satisfying and filling, followed by applesauce, and the apple juice was the least filling and satisfying of the three. It took research subjects more time to eat the apples. Juice was consumed eleven times faster than the apples, and four times quicker than the applesauce.

ESSENTIAL VITAMINS

Vitamins and minerals are essential *micronutrients,* needed in very small amounts to keep our bodies functioning properly. Most people get enough of the thirteen vitamins and the necessary minerals, such as iron and calcium, when they eat a well-balanced diet. The catch is that many people still don't eat a balanced diet.

People with diabetes who are cutting their calorie intake to below 1,200 calories per day to lose weight or control blood sugars are frequently advised to take vitamin and mineral supplements because it's difficult to meet the average daily requirements with severely restricted food choices. However, few dietitians recommend diets below 1,200 calories. Some advise people who are restricting their food intake to take one multivitamin tablet per day, simply as insurance against not getting adequate supplies of all vitamins in their food.

Consult your doctor before you begin taking large doses of vitamin supplements. Tell your doctor what vitamins you take, just as you tell him or her about your medications. Vitamins are foods, not medicines. Megavitamin supplements will not cure diabetes and they are not a substitute for nutritious food, medical treatment, or physical activity, although supplements can be helpful in some cases. The use of vitamin supplements remains controversial, although the use of certain vitamins is more accepted now than in years past.

A survey of vitamin-related research by Daniel E. Baker, Pharm.D., and R. Keith Campbell of Washington State University, published in the magazine *Diabetes Educator* in 1992 concluded: "Some degree of supplementation with certain vitamins (e.g., vitamin C and vitamin E) and minerals (e.g., magnesium) may be beneficial to prevent long-term complications of diabetes. Daily supplements of vitamin C, vitamin E, and magnesium ultimately may do some good, and unless the patient has a severe renal dysfunction, probably will do no harm to the person with diabetes."

A few vitamins, such as niacin, taken for other health conditions can actually *raise* blood sugar levels; their use should be closely monitored in people with diabetes. Niacin is sometimes prescribed at a level of 50 to 100 mg per day, to lower fat and triglyceride levels. Because they can raise blood sugar, do not begin taking niacin supplements before checking with the doctor who is treating your diabetes.

People with diabetes often have unusually low levels of certain vitamins, particularly two antioxidant vitamins, vitamin C and vitamin E. The American Diabetes Association cites "theoretical reasons" in favor of antioxidant supplements, but does not recommend them because they say the benefits have not been confirmed.

Vitamin C levels in the blood are low in people with diabetes compared to people without diabetes who have similar diets. The reason for this is unclear. A large study of the diets of Finnish and Dutch men over several decades showed a relationship between low vitamin C intake and glucose intolerance, a precursor to Type 2 diabetes. Supplementation with vitamin C is believed to help prevent or reduce incidences of some complications, such as cataracts and nerve disorders. One study showed that 1,400 mg per day of vitamin C improved the results of glycosylated hemoglobin tests. On the downside, vitamin C supplementation can throw off the results of a urinary test. Vitamin C is found in many fruits and vegetables, including citrus fruits, berries, tomatoes, lettuce, green peppers, potatoes, and cantaloupe, and it's sometimes used as an additive in other foods. Vitamin C and vitamin E are antioxidants, which can help repair cell structures damaged by oxidation and high blood sugar.

Vitamin E has well-known beneficial effects on the heart and the circulatory system. Assuring that vitamin E intake is at least up to daily requirements can reduce the chance of complications involving the heart and blood vessels, including cataracts and other problems involving the small blood vessels of the eyes. Adequate vitamin E may inhibit the production of a blood clotting chemical called thromboxane, which can damage blood vessels. Vitamin E is found in wheat germ, whole grain cereals, soybean and canola oil, green leafy vegetables, and egg yolks.

Supplements of antioxidants at reasonable levels may help you, but it's probably better to get most of your antioxidants directly from food. Food contains complicated mixtures of not only vitamins and minerals, but also thousands of other beneficial substances that activate various processes in the body. Vitamin supplements are chemically different from food, and they don't contain fiber. You may not want to place all your faith in individual supplements. All the antioxidants work best as a sort of biochemical team—what Lester Packer, Ph.D., of the University of California calls the "antioxidant network."

Magnesium, a mineral concentrated in the organs and skeleton, is rarely depleted in the general population. However, some recent studies have found that as many as 25 percent of people with diabetes have a magnesium deficiency. Magnesium is believed to play a role in the release of insulin from the pancreas and in blood pressure control. Magnesium may be depleted by high blood sugar, and diuretics such as coffee. Significantly, some low-calorie diets given to people with diabetes to help them lose weight may not meet the recommended daily allowance for magnesium. If your magnesium levels are low, supplements at the recommended daily allowance may improve glycemic control. Magnesium supplements are *not* recommended for people with kidney problems. Foods containing magnesium include spinach, broccoli, whole grain and bran cereals, cashew nuts, peanuts, almonds, soybeans, whole wheat, rice, dried fruits, dry beans, peas, potatoes, milk, shrimp, fish, and even chocolate. Almost all unprocessed foods contain some magnesium, but food processing depletes it.

Lots of claims are made for another mineral, chromium, which in the chromium picolinate form may increase insulin sensitivity and slightly lower blood sugar. Chromium is a mineral needed by the body in tiny amounts, but even those amounts are difficult to get from eating a typical diet as processed foods have basically been robbed of chromium. Brewer's yeast, organ meats, mushrooms, and broccoli are good natural sources but scarce in most diets. Taking between 200 to 1,000 micrograms of chromium per day has been shown in some tests to slightly lower blood sugar, HbA1c levels, and blood fat levels. A study conducted in China on people newly diagnosed with Type 2 diabetes showed significant reductions after supplementation at the rate of 1,000 micrograms per day for two months, and greater reductions at four months. Lesser levels of improvement were achieved with daily supplements of 200 micrograms. Yehuda Handelsman, M.D., a Los Angeles doctor who specializes in diabetes, recommends chromium picolinate supplements, 200 micrograms twice a day as part of an overall program that includes diet, exercise, and medications. Chromium picolinate should be taken under a doctor's supervision, with careful monitoring of blood glucose levels to determine if levels of diabetes medication or insulin should be adjusted as a result. Some nutritionists recommend a supplement containing chromium picolinate and magnesium for people with Type 2 diabetes. Vanadium is another trace mineral that may prove to increase insulin sensitivity. The amounts of these minerals required by the body are quite small, and deficiencies are difficult to even measure. Zinc supplements have been touted as a way to improve insulin utilization, but this has not been proven (although zinc has a general role in healing).

There is some evidence that folic acid, one of the B vitamins, can aid in preventing vascular disease in people with diabetes. Alpha-lipoic acid has reduced fasting glucose levels in some studies, and gamma-linolenic acid (evening primrose oil) has been shown to improve nerve function in animal studies. The omega-3 fatty acids found in fish and canola oil lower triglyceride levels but have little effect on glucose levels, according to recent research.

MOTIVATION

Strategies to change eating patterns vary by individual. Thinking this through will take some brain work, and perhaps a bit of trial and error. You can change your eating style, but you must keep yourself motivated, especially in the beginning.

Because making food choices can raise questions, you may work best with a dietitian, who will guide you and answer your questions as you go along. You may be a person who is *only* able to change your eating patterns with the help of a group such as Weight Watchers, which can offer lots of positive reinforcement and group support. Or you may be able to wake up one morning, decide to change, and pull it off single-handedly.

Changing your eating style is a long-haul proposition. Think of it as planning for a series of small vacations. Most things you'll be able to anticipate; planning will help you enjoy yourself. On the other hand, no matter how carefully you plan, you won't be able to anticipate every little twist and turn in the road.

It's important to set both short-term and long-term goals for yourself, and to move forward at your own pace. Don't rush yourself. If you achieve a goal, treat yourself with small gifts and rewards, such as a trip to the movies, or simply tell someone about your success. Don't set unrealistically high goals for yourself, such as losing 20 pounds a week, and then fall into the oldest diet trap of all—feeling guilty, and hating yourself because you can't do the impossible. Remember that a little improvement every day or every week is preferable to none. The idea is to always make progress, not to achieve perfection. If you can get it right about 80 percent of the time, many professionals say you're on the right track. First you learn, then you use what you've learned to make sensible and flavorful food choices that fit into your life and even make it more exciting.

Changing your eating style may be easier if you haven't already tried a lot of crash diets and fallen into the mind-set that you can't possibly succeed with any diet. Most crash diets are so restrictive that the great majority of people who attempt them fail. However, *anyone* can slowly change her eating style. Even grizzled diet veterans can succeed, especially if they are motivated by something such as controlling their blood sugar or improving the course of their lives. Sometimes newcomers to these concepts, such as men, can even do better.

Your chances for success increase if you have a strong motive for changing your eating habits, such as seeing a favorite overweight relative or friend (who may even have diabetes) barely survive a heart attack, or suffer complications. Being diagnosed with diabetes may be motivation enough for you. Psychological research has shown that you're most likely to change your behavior if you have a good, strong reason to do so.

If you're looking for a way to motivate yourself, a desire to improve your health for the rest of your life may be sufficient incentive to change.

THE JOY OF COOKING

Unfortunately, it's easy to fall into the TV dinner diet trap. This is the trap where you eat the TV dinner, but don't really feel full, so you eat some more.

If you cook for yourself, according to registered dietitian Diane Woods, you're often ahead of the game. If you cook, you have control over *all* the ingredients in your meals. You can substitute healthier ingredients, use less sugar, control the portions that you eat, and experience the fun of actively moving around the kitchen with the fragrant smell of good food in the air and perhaps some relaxing music on the radio. Cooking a quick meal can take as little as ten minutes of your time. Many recent good cookbooks emphasize quick, delicious, easy-to-prepare meals. You may not be able to cook every day and every night, but you *can* spend ten to fifteen minutes every now and then preparing your own meals, and savoring the experience.

If you eat slowly and relish each bite, and if you give yourself permission to enjoy the experience of eating, you may find yourself eating a bit less food, but enjoying it more. Gourmet chef Julia Child recently observed that many Americans think of food much as they think of medicine, rather than seeing a meal as the sensual experience and social catalyst that it ought to be. For goodness sake, enjoy your food.

In the minds of many overweight people, the guilt associated with eating has taken the pleasure away. No matter what your weight, consider it important that you give yourself permission to eat slowly, chewing each bite a few times. Try to spend at least twenty minutes eating each meal. Believe it or not, this helps change destructive eating patterns. The nineteenth-century nutritionist Horace Fletcher recommended that every person chew each bite of food thirty-two times, since that is the number of teeth we have. Fletcher's advice may be overstated, but taking a moment to savor each mouthful is a good idea simply because you'll taste every bite of your food and it will take you longer to eat it. A well-known medical doctor has a trick that works for him—since the first and last bites are always the best, he allows himself one and only one bite of the richest, gooeyest, most fattening desserts. And then he stops.

Be your own friend in self-management, especially when it comes to food. Working to like—or love—yourself and to cherish and celebrate each small success will cause the positive aspects of your changes in eating style to compound. But become your own worst enemy and focus only on your mistakes, and you'll find that the guilt, depression, and horrible feelings of failure will also compound. Work to forgive yourself if you slip, because you are human. But work just as hard to reward yourself when you succeed.

Changing your eating style may create battles within your family. Know who your friends are in this area, as well as those who might want to sabotage your meal plan. In the battle of the bulge, your first mission is to take care of yourself. Situations that pose risks for some people include being depressed, frustrated, or under stress; having a normal schedule suddenly disrupted; being pressured for time; feeling deprived or left out; or attending various social events with family or friends.

"Diabetes is such an individual thing. For instance, we all react so differently to different foods," one woman says. "I've learned that I have to watch myself. When I'm not in a good spot, that's when I'm weak. Sometimes, there are people out there who will try to sabotage you."

Some of your so-called friends may say, "Oh, you can get away with eating an extra piece of wedding cake just this one time." If you reply that you're on a diet, they may try to pull you off the wagon. However, if you simply refuse the second piece of cake with a polite, "No thank you, I'm full," the discussion should end because few people will try to give you food when you don't want it. A 1990 study of women who lost weight and maintained the weight loss showed that the women successful in losing weight and keeping it off devised strategies and plans to lose weight that fit their lives. The most successful women had a tendency to confront rather than avoid problems and to distract themselves by exercise, work, or shopping, rather than by eating, smoking, sleeping, or wishing the problem would magically disappear. They were more likely to exercise and less likely to try "quick fix" solutions such as diet pills or fad diets. Women who maintained their weight loss allowed themselves to eat their favorite foods occasionally in moderation and were a little more likely to have support from friends or family members.

Bring your family members into the picture, if you can. They can help a lot, not by lecturing incessantly about what you should and shouldn't eat, but by giving you a pat on the back when you achieve a personal goal. If your family members are supportive, tell them when you lose your first 2 or 3 pounds, or whenever you feel that you have accomplished a little something. If you're comfortable doing so, ask for a reasonable amount of help when you feel other people might support your efforts.

When you make a shopping list and go to the market, be sure to buy healthy, nutritious foods such as fresh vegetables and fruits. Keep healthy foods in your home at all times. If needed, make a special list to get started; you may even wish to make a trip to the farmer's market or a health food store. Integrate the foods into your life that you know are healthy and nutritious, and that will help you control your blood sugar. Buy whole grain foods, fresh fruits and vegetables, fish, low-fat milk, diet sodas, low-fat ice cream, sugar substitutes, and whatever else is on your list. Unprocessed foods are generally healthier than processed foods. Make a list. Planning will help you succeed.

PRACTICAL TIPS

Here are a few quick practical tips to help you change your eating style and control your weight and blood sugar:

- Spread calories around throughout the day, and don't eat all your carbohydrates at the same meal.
- Eat salad first, then wait half an hour to eat the rest of the meal.
- Make yourself aware of portion sizes for particular items. This will give you better control at home and when eating out. On exchange lists, for instance, one serving of rice is ⅓ cup. If you eat at a Chinese restaurant, where a normal serving is 1 cup of rice, ask for less rice. Portion size means ½ cup of yams, 1¼ cups of strawberries, or half an apple. How do you eat half an apple? Dip the uneaten half in citrus juice to stop oxidation or prevent the apple from turning brown.
- Unsweeten sweet foods. With canned fruit, pour out the juice;

if packed in syrup, rinse it off the fruit. Try sugar substitutes such as Equal or aspartame in place of sucrose.

- Satisfy your hunger by snacking on high-fiber, low-calorie items such as salads and vegetables. Vegetables have fewer calories than fruits, and fruits have more fiber than fruit juice. Graham crackers, whole wheat bread, and bran cereal are all high-fiber snacks.

- Read food labels. Some foods labeled No Fat, such as no-fat mayonnaise, are made with carbohydrates substituted for fat—the extra carbohydrates may add up to an additional serving of starch or fruit. Reading food labels will tell you much of what you need to know to work a particular food into your eating plans.

- When eating out, eat half the entrée portion (which is often too large); request doggie bags to take the rest home for another meal, or request a half-serving. An alternative is splitting part of your dinner with your dinner companion, which also saves money.

PRACTICAL TRICKS

Here are a few more quick tips that might help you cope with the psychic ups and downs of adopting a new eating style:

- Make it really easy to eat healthy foods and difficult to eat unhealthy foods. Keep fresh fruits and vegetables handy. Remove temptation from your refrigerator or workplace. Leave yourself written orders on the refrigerator to eat nutritious snacks when you're hungry. Hide the cookies or cookie jar. If you can't stop with one, don't eat the first one. Ask family members to work with you.

HOLIDAY DIET TIPS

Among all the holidays that we celebrate with food feasts, the winter holidays are sometimes most perilous for people with diabetes. In some families, the main holiday event is a big meal of high-fat, high-calorie food. The holidays are also stressful times, and many people handle stress by nibbling on food. Plan ahead. Planning can help keep your holiday eating under control, and can be helpful in special situations involving the perils of rich, overabundant food, notes Therese Farrell, R.D.

Just maintaining your current weight is often the best goal during the holidays. Set reasonable weight-loss goals, and don't beat yourself up for too long if you slip, or gain an extra pound. Before Thanksgiving dinner, remember the last Thanksgiving that you overate, and how bloated and uncomfortable you felt afterward. In all cases, *moderation* is advised, because almost anything can be enjoyed in small amounts.

Here are a few tips for handling some of the perilous situations you're likely to encounter over the holidays:

- Eat what you like, but take smaller portions of foods that you know are rich, and eat them slowly to savor each mouthful.
- Do some additional exercise or physical activity to compensate for the extra food you may eat. Going for a short walk after dinner will help you relax and lower blood sugars.
- If you have a choice, choose low-fat items over high-fat ones, and skip the food items you might not really need or want, such as extra butter on bread.
- Keep a supply of light foods such as fruits, vegetables, and prepared salads on hand for eating between parties and when you're on the go.
- Plan how much food you will eat at a party, and tell your significant other about your plans if that will help. Snack before the party, arrive fashionably late, and bring only a small plate to the buffet table.
- Give healthy gifts such as fruit baskets or low-calorie cookbooks rather than boxes of candy.

- If you receive a high-calorie gift, exercise your generosity and give away that box of candy to someone else, or even to a needy family or homeless person who truly needs the calories.
- If you're throwing a party, try to make it a potluck, and provide suggestions for low-fat, low-calorie dishes if people ask.
- If you're baking cookies or other treats, experiment with lower portions of fat ingredients, or substitute some artificial sugar for real sugar. Cooking does involve some beneficial exercise, but try to control your tasting. Give away any extra baked items as soon as possible, or if giving them as gifts, store them in sealed containers and place them in hard-to-get-to locations to keep the Munching Demon at bay.
- If you drink alcohol, drink in moderation and avoid sugary mixed drinks. When you drink, eat a little something too.
- If you ruin your game plan by overindulging, admit your mistake, then immediately forgive yourself and get back to work. Don't wait until New Year's Day to resume watching what you eat.

◦ Use smaller plates to make portions appear larger.

◦ Don't reward yourself with food. Instead, call a favorite relative or old friend and chat, buy yourself a bouquet of flowers, rent a sexy video, or treat yourself to a day trip to a museum or the zoo. The same recommendations apply to people who punish themselves by eating more food.

◦ Instead of eating, exercise. Even just a short walk around the block will help get your mind off eating and put your feet back on the ground.

◦ Don't assign moral values to foods. Celery sticks, chocolate éclairs, eggs Benedict, or any other food can be reduced to its numerical essence, calories. If you eat the "bad" fruitcake in a moment of weakness, simply calculate the calories, add them to your list, and get back on track as soon as possible.

- ✦ Don't beat yourself up for more than twenty-four hours if you slip and happen to eat something forbidden. Forgive yourself, slap your wrist, vow to do better, and move on with your life.

DIET PILLS AND SURGERY

Most of us would like to go to a doctor and get a magic pill or have a little operation that makes all our problems go away. In a society that values instant gratification, diet pills may seem like the answer. Diet pills work as long as you take them, but they are not a panacea for losing weight. Diet pills containing amphetamines have had a sinister reputation for years, due to side effects that can include psychosis. The newer diet pills are believed to be more benign, even though their use is restricted in many states to a period of weeks. The new diet pills do suppress appetite, and people do lose weight, but they gain the weight back again when they stop taking the pills.

Many diet pills typically produce an initial loss of 20 to 25 pounds, after which you feel good and gain back 10 to 15 pounds, to wind up with a 10- to 12-pound loss. This pattern applies to people on the once-fashionable Phen-Fen diet or Redux as well as other substances that can result in weight loss, such as Prozac and cigarettes. A few new drugs target the seriously obese, but these medications are not suitable for all people and should be used only under a doctor's supervision. One, sibutramine (Meridia), was approved in 1997 and prolongs the "full" feeling you have after eating a meal. Another new drug, orlistat (Xenical) was effective in a study of 254 obese patients with Type 2 diabetes, who lost more weight (6.2 percent of their body weight versus 4.3 percent) than the control group and also lowered the amount of medication they required. Xenical is a lipase inhibitor, blocking the absorption of fat in the intestine, but also unfortunately blocking the absorption of fat-soluble vitamins such as Vitamins A, D, E, and K. The drug is recommended only for people who are very obese. Both Meridia and Xenical must be taken indefinitely, and like all drugs, they have side effects. Side effects of Meridia can include constipation, dry mouth, insomnia, and increased blood pressure. Orlistat can cause oily, liquid, or loose stools; flatulence; and abdominal pain. If you do take these medications, remember that any weight-loss program is most effective when combined with lasting changes in diet, exercise habits, and lifestyle.

If you took diet pills such as the once popular Phen-Fen diet pill combination or Redux, your doctor should check you for signs of damage to your heart or lungs as a precaution, because these drugs have been shown to produce heart valve damage in some patients. An echocardiogram test, which is painless, can aid your doctor in locating heart valve problems or in giving you a clean bill of health. If you do have heart valve damage, you may need to receive antibiotics before teeth cleanings, tooth removal, and a few other similar procedures as a precaution.

Medical science has begun to view obesity as a condition that needs to be treated for life. Since pills are a quick fix with temporary benefits and unknown long-term effects, think about changing your eating style slowly enough to have a lasting beneficial impact on weight, and a lowering effect on blood sugar.

In very extreme cases, surgery may be employed to aid weight loss. Weight-loss surgery basically reduces the capacity of the stomach to hold food. The two main types of weight-loss surgery are gastric bypass surgery, which reroutes food to the small intestine, and restriction surgery, which restricts the amount of food in the stomach. Any surgery is risky, and infections can occur from leaks in the stomach or intestines.

Most people lose a lot of weight after these types of surgery, which usually causes glucose and blood pressure levels to drop as a result of the weight loss. According to guidelines from the American Obesity Association, stomach surgery is a medical option when a person is at extremely high health risk from being overweight. People with eating disorders or unstable medical or mental conditions are not good candidates for these surgeries.

Although the benefits of such surgeries are obvious, complications can include the stomach stretching to allow more food in after surgery. Staples placed in the stomach can leak. Vomiting is the most frequent side effect, but lactose intolerance, ulcers, vitamin deficiencies, mineral deficiencies, and even malnutrition can occur.

Although drugs and surgery can help some people, for most, a basic strategy of healthy diet, regular exercise, and perhaps medications is the preferred route to good control.

SUGAR, SALT, AND MORE

People with diabetes are sometimes advised to decrease their intake of sugar, dietary cholesterol, salt, and even alcohol.

ABOUT ARTIFICIAL SWEETENERS

Since sugars are pure carbohydrates that move quickly into the bloodstream to become blood sugar, some dietitians recommend the moderate use of calorie-free sugar substitutes to cut calories and carbohydrates. Artificial sweeteners allow people to reduce calories while still enjoying sweetened foods. Diet sodas, jams, jellies, and chewing gum flavored with aspartame will not affect blood sugar; substituting these items for those made with real sugar can be helpful for people with diabetes. Artificial sugars such as saccharin, acesulfame K, sucralose, and aspartame may be used to sweeten beverages such as coffee and tea, and may sometimes be substituted for sugar in recipes. A much smaller quantity of these products is necessary for sweetness because they are all highly concentrated. Saccharin, for instance, sold under the brand names Sweet 'N Low, Sucaryl, Sugar Twin, Sweet Magic, and Zero-Cal, is 375 times sweeter than regular sugar, and can be used as a substitute in regular cooking by most people, although pregnant women are advised to avoid it. Acesulfame-K, sold as Sweet One and Swiss Sweet, is 200 times sweeter than sucrose and can be used in cooking. A new sweetener, sucralose, sold under the brand name Splenda, is manufactured from sugar by rearranging sugar molecules. Splenda is not digested in the body. Some 600 times sweeter than sugar, Splenda can be used as a sweetener and in baking. It was originally available only to people with diabetes. Aspartame, sold under the brand names Equal, Sweetmate, and Spoonfuls, is 180 times sweeter than sucrose, but is not an acceptable substitute for baking since it loses its sweetening effect when heated. Diet sodas and other drinks containing aspartame are often considered "free foods"—their use in exchange list diets is unrestricted because the calorie content is low (nutritional content is also low). If you use artificial sweeteners, use them in moderation. Five to ten packets per day or less is an acceptable amount. Some controversy exists over the sweetener products, saccharin being the oldest of the three. The U.S. Food and Drug Administration doesn't consider aspartame harmful because it doesn't cause cancer in lab animals. But high amounts of saccharin have apparently caused cancer in lab animals (this is printed as a warning on the labels of saccharin products), although it is unclear whether this research applies to humans.

If you have a sweet tooth and want to keep sweetness in your meals, cut back on the amount of sugar that you use. Cut the amount of sugar added to recipes a bit each time you make them, or substitute nutmeg, cinnamon, almond extract, or vanilla for sugar. Fresh fruits are sweet snacks, with the added health benefit of fiber.

ABOUT CHOLESTEROL

Much confusion exists about cholesterol because high cholesterol levels in the blood are a well-publicized precursor to heart attacks. Cholesterol is a form of fat that contributes to the development of such sex hormones as estrogen and testosterone, and it's needed by cell membranes. Most of the cholesterol you need to survive is manufactured in your liver. *Dietary cholesterol* is present in all animal products, particularly those containing saturated fats. Saturated fats elevate your blood, or serum, cholesterol. The average American eats food containing 400 mg of cholesterol per day, but needs to consume almost none. Cholesterol levels typically rise a bit in the winter and fall a bit in the summer. Cholesterol is tested as part of a lipid profile, one of the tests covered in chapter 10 on laboratory tests. A desirable cholesterol level is less than 200.

ABOUT SODIUM

Sodium, or salt, is another essential element, and it's a big factor in fluid retention, which can add weight. Although in ancient times salt was so scarce that it was used as a substitute for money, most of us today have way too much salt in our diets. Americans typically consume 6,000 to 10,000 mg per day, much more than we need. Sodium is freely sprinkled over most TV dinners, snack foods, hot dogs, and canned soups as a preservative and flavor enhancer. Health authorities recommend between 2,400 and 3,000 mg of sodium per day for most people. The American Diabetes Association's 1995 clinical practice guidelines recommend a maximum of 2,400 mg per day for people with mild to moderate high blood pressure, and 2,000 mg or less for people with kidney complications and high blood pressure. Sodium is now listed on food labels, expressed in milligrams and as a percentage of the 2,400 mg recommendation. People with high blood pressure or other complications of diabetes are often advised to cut their salt intake to normal or below-normal levels to help lower their blood pressure. As a rule of thumb, look for 500 mg or less of sodium *per serving* in processed food items.

ABOUT ALCOHOL

Alcohol lowers blood sugar, but it does contain empty calories, which should be included in calorie counting. Some doctors believe that it's okay to have a drink or two every day because of alcohol's relaxing qualities and because alcohol raises the "good," or HDL, cholesterol. If you are taking medication for your diabetes, talk to your doctor before you drink, since drinking can interfere with the action of some medications. Alcohol increases your risk of experiencing hypoglycemia or low blood sugar, so prepare for this by having a quick-acting carbohydrate snack on hand if you drink. Make sure the mixed drinks you consume don't contain extra sugar—shy away from those cute, sugary tropical-type mixed drinks that come decorated with little cherries and umbrellas. Don't drink without eating something, either.

CHECK YOUR MEDICINES

It's normally not a problem, but many prescription and over-the-counter medicines contain a bit of sweetener to give tablets a more palatable taste. Even those labeled sugar free should be checked to assure that they don't contain dextrose, fructose, or sorbitol, which are forms of sugar. Get in the habit of reading the labels of medicines as well as foods. People who are ill or under stress should monitor their blood sugar levels frequently; during those situations, avoid medicines that contain a bit of sugar. Some medicines also contain alcohol, which you'll discover when you read the label.

YES, YOU CAN SUCCEED

When you bring about a change in your eating style, you can help yourself control your blood sugar levels and perhaps lose weight. Consult a registered dietitian or a reliable nutritional consultant and follow her recommendations. Select a personal approach to eating. A balanced diet is always best, one that assures you of adequate nutrients of all types. When combined with a more physically active lifestyle, the subject of the next chapter, changing your eating style will dramatically change the way you feel today, and help give you the benefit of better long-term health tomorrow.

Chapter 8

EXERCISE

How You Profit from a More Physically Active Lifestyle

~

BECOMING MORE PHYSICALLY ACTIVE IS ANOTHER LIFESTYLE CHOICE THAT WILL HELP lower and control your blood sugar. This aspect of self-management may also help you to lose weight and achieve better health. Physical activity comes in many forms, of course, and all deliver both physical and emotional benefits. Your medical doctor or an exercise physiologist may work with you in developing a program of activity or exercise, particularly if it's a dramatic change from your current lifestyle. Becoming more physically active may involve a strategy to work more physical activity into your life, or even to join sports clubs or exercise classes. Any activity that you choose should be enjoyable—and sustainable—for you. Some special precautions exist, particularly for older people or people with medical complications. As with all aspects of self-management, a new physically active lifestyle should first be tailored to fit your interests.

The two major lifestyle changes that can control your blood sugar are changes in your eating style and increased physical activity. Every person needs to use his body, particularly the larger groups of muscles and the lungs, a little bit every day. Physical activity has long been recognized as a key to good health and well-being. A study of Harvard University graduates published in *The New England Journal of Medicine* claimed that for every hour most people spend exercising, they actually add an hour to their lives.

"No less than two hours a day should be devoted to exercise," declared the third U.S. president, Thomas Jefferson, a Virginia gentleman farmer who was physically active until his death in 1826. More than 150 years later, President John F. Kennedy cited Jefferson when he urged Americans to become more physically active by observing, "If the man who wrote the Declaration of Independence, was secretary of state, and twice president, could give it two hours, our children can give it ten or fifteen minutes."

New benefits of exercise are still being discovered. But physical activity should be enjoyable, and not hazardous; begin adopting changes slowly and don't overdo it. Finding a physical activity that you enjoy can be a way to have fun, and firm up your body in the process.

The doctor who treats your diabetes may write you an exercise prescription or refer you to an exercise physiologist, who specializes in the effects of physical activity on the body. The person you see should help you develop a program that matches your physical needs with your interests and abilities. Any exercise prescription will involve a choice of physical activity, and recommendations for both the intensity and frequency of exercise. Many exercise physiologists are also certified diabetes educators who can explain how particular exercises affect your blood sugar. This is not usually true of personal trainers at health clubs, who often have degrees in physical education but are not up to speed on diabetes.

Before making any exercise recommendations, your doctor or exercise physiologist must consider your medical history as well as any complications that you may have. Most important, this person should look at how you have been doing recently with blood glucose control. Heart disease risk factors, physical characteristics, age, weight, physical condition, and the results of pertinent diagnostic tests should all be taken into account. Also considered should be your personal lifestyle, any limitations that you have, and the medications that you take. For instance, medicines called beta blockers, often prescribed for cardiac problems, can slow your heart's normal response to exercise and cover up low blood sugar.

Some medical tests are useful before beginning any program of physical activity. The American Diabetes Association recommends that people over thirty-five years of age have a treadmill test, which allows a physician to gauge your exercise tolerance to see if your body can handle additional physical stress. Electrocardiograms are frequently given. A stress test is given if you've had diabetes for more than ten years. Ideally, your doctor or exercise physiologist should recommend a safe, enjoyable program that can be sustained, and be of continuing benefit to you.

Always check with your doctor before beginning any new exercise program. Special limits on exercise apply to people with diabetes who have complications such as macrovascular or microvascular disease. Exercises that are most appropriate to people with complications are included in chapter 15.

BIG BENEFITS

Most programs of self-management involve a certain level of physical activity or regular exercise. Exercise has many benefits when done carefully and regularly.

If exercise were a pill, every doctor alive would prescribe it to patients with Type 2 diabetes because of its miraculous effects. Along with great short-term and long-term physical and mental benefits, exercise has almost no detrimental side effects if properly done. This is why a medical doctor's recommendations for exercise are often called an exercise prescription. Exercise is known as the "other insulin" because of its direct, beneficial impact on lowering blood sugar.

Your muscles use at least 95 percent of the glucose that your body produces. If you don't use your muscles very much, they don't use much glucose. Inactivity is part of the reason that glucose backs up in your blood, elevating blood sugar. It stands to reason that using your muscles more often will cause them to utilize more glucose, and lower blood sugar. Aerobic exercise will *always* produce an immediate drop in your blood sugar.

Since blood sugar levels rise and fall, the best times to get physically active or to exercise are usually when blood sugars are the highest. This is frequently about an hour after meals, and first thing in the morning. Blood sugar testing at various times of the day will tell you when your blood sugar levels are highest. Whenever your blood sugar is high, that's the ideal time to do some physical activity.

HOW EXERCISE WORKS

Perhaps the most obvious benefit of exercise is its ability to accelerate weight loss. When you become more physically active, you burn up more calories and use insulin more efficiently. You also build up your overall health and vigor. Exercise makes your heart pump faster, which strengthens your heart and all the other muscles that you use. As you engage in physical activity, your body burns fat and cholesterol. Your muscle tone improves, reducing any muscle atrophy that has occurred. Following an exercise program also helps prevent the onset of diabetes—something you may want to discuss with your children, grandchildren, or other relatives if diabetes runs in your family.

Physical activity will help you improve the quality of your life. This is partially because exercise combats depression, and relieves physical and emotional stress. Strenuous exercise releases happy chemicals called beta endorphins into your bloodstream, chemicals that create euphoria and relieve pain. Even moderate exercise causes your body to release mood-altering chemical substances, which perk up your spirit.

Physical activity helps the body to utilize glucose. For most people, a half hour of moderate physical activity will cause blood sugar levels to drop 20 to 25 percent. This drop is due to greater burning of sugars by muscle cells during exercise, a lesser production of glucose within the body, and the creation of new insulin receptors on your cell membranes. If your blood sugar levels are too high, exercise will make them drop, sometimes for more than twenty-four hours after one exercise session.

A FEW WELL-KNOWN BENEFITS OF EXERCISE

Benefits for the Body

- Increased insulin sensitivity lowers blood sugar
- Burns calories to help weight loss
- Burns off harmful fats and cholesterol
- Lowers blood pressure
- Strengthens heart and lungs
- Increases muscle strength and endurance
- Increases bone density
- Decreases sensation of physical pain
- Improves reaction time
- Improves central nervous system function
- Reduces physical stress

Benefits for the Mind

- You feel better immediately
- Your self-confidence improves
- Your body image improves
- Helps control depression
- Increases mental flexibility
- Improves memory
- Reduces emotional stress

When combined with changes in eating style, physical activity results in even better control of blood sugar. Even if you completely change your style of eating, even greater weight loss, greater insulin sensitivity, and lower blood sugar will be achieved when dieting is done along with exercise. Exercise helps your body burn fat alone, rather than the combination of fats, proteins, and lean muscle tissue that are burned by simply dieting. Weight-bearing exercise reduces the risk of osteoporosis in women. Exercise relieves stress, distracts you from your problems, stimulates your brain, and reduces mental depression by both giving you an immediate psychological lift and by releasing chemicals such as serotonin and norepinephrine into the brain. All these things are beneficial to your physical, mental, and emotional health.

OBESITY

Obesity and being overweight are serious health problems in industrialized countries. According to the U.S. Centers for Disease Control, approximately 24 percent of all Americans have a completely sedentary lifestyle, while 54 percent engage in less than thirty minutes of moderate physical activity most days of the week. Excessive body weight can almost always be controlled by a regular program of exercise and diet.

Obesity is defined as "an excessive accumulation of body fat," specifically, fat levels greater than 25 percent of total body weight in men and 30 percent in women. *Overweight,* a more general term, means that a person's total weight is greater than a statistical average, even though that weight could include a substantial percentage of muscle, which weighs more than fat. Of the two conditions, obesity is more hazardous to your health. Whether or not you have diabetes, obesity is harmful because the extra weight puts a greater burden on the body's normal operations, increasing the risk of heart disease, high blood pressure, hemorrhoids, hiatal hernia, arthritis, and cancer.

Continuing obesity can increase the likelihood of all the known complications of diabetes, because over time it multiplies the negative effects of high blood sugar on the body. According to Dr. Claudia Graham, a certified diabetes educator in Los Angeles who has a doctorate in exercise science, the presence of excessive fat tissue in the body is harmful because it blocks the beneficial effects of insulin. Dr. Graham's ideas about exercise may be found in *The Diabetes Sports and Exercise Book,* cowritten with June Biermann and Barbara Toohey.

THE SEDENTARY LIFE

Sadly, the average American spends almost five hours a day watching television, according to the Center for Science in the Public Interest. Television watching is almost always a passive, sedentary activity, one that requires the viewer to sit and stare for a long time in one direction—a somewhat unnatural thing for the muscles of the human body to do. Television watching is often accompanied by sweet or fat-laden snacks. Commercials exhort you to buy more junk food, fast food, beer, and sugary carbonated drinks. Watching television affects your brain waves, which slow into an alpha state, causing your metabolism to slow down.

If you watch a lot of television, consider missing one or two shows and devoting that time to physical activity. You could substitute an exercise class or a leisurely stroll around the neighborhood for your least favorite programs. You might videotape the programs that you miss. If you can't miss even one program, could you move an exercise machine or stationary bicycle into the room and do something with your body while you watch?

Every person's physical prowess declines with age. Research has shown that between the ages of thirty and seventy, flexibility typically declines by 20 to 30 percent, muscle mass declines by 25 to 30 percent, work capacity declines by 25 to 30 percent, and bone mass declines by 25 to 30 percent in women and 15 to 20 percent in men. This is the basic bad news about aging. But consider the benefits of exercise: it strengthens the cardiovascular system, the muscles, the joint structure, and bone composition. The good news is that even a moderate amount of exercise has a correlation with longevity. Most of us know individuals who remain active long past their prime, with minds and hearts fully engaged in their lives and interests. It's not a coincidence that most of these people have led physically active lives.

As one becomes more physically active, the muscles firm and the body becomes slender and fit. Physical activity improves muscle strength and flexibility, and lowers the blood pressure. Cardiovascular function improves; fats and glucose in the bloodstream burn away. For the person with diabetes, blood sugar swings become less frequent and dramatic, and therefore less harmful. You may need less medication or insulin when you incorporate physical activity into your life. And a few pounds may melt away.

When you choose to become more physically active, you empower yourself a little bit more each day.

FITNESS

A physically active lifestyle doesn't mean you have to spend every spare minute in exercise classes, dressed in a designer sweatsuit, waving your arms and legs in a furious, flapping, sweat-drenched workout. It doesn't mean that you must suddenly begin jogging 10 miles to work, or lifting weights like a young Arnold Schwarzenegger. Fitness involves you as you are. If you add more physical activity to your life, you will become more physically fit. Selecting an activity that you can enjoy, or at least tolerate, is important because the primary obstacles to exercise are not physical, but psychological.

If you wish to enjoy the known benefits of physical activity, including better blood sugar control and the loss of weight, what you are shooting for is a healthy level of physical fitness. This is a level of activity you can sustain that is adequate to help control blood sugar. According to Dr. Graham, you do not need a level of fitness adequate to participate in team sports, or the stamina to compete in a 10-mile run and not embarrass yourself. Health-related fitness is all you really need to control blood sugar, and it's enough to help you lose weight.

Think for a while about what you enjoy and don't enjoy doing. Choose physical activities that you personally enjoy, whether or not you think of those activities as exercise. Would it suit you to integrate some exercise into your workday, to walk up the stairs to your office rather than taking the elevator, or to park a few blocks away so that you can walk to and from the office? Would you enjoy spending more time sight-seeing, traveling, or playing with your children or grandchildren?

Are you the solitary type, who would enjoy becoming more active outdoors—chopping wood, shoveling snow, working in your yard, or tending a community garden? Could you do more housework yourself, or do it more frequently? Could you find a frisky little dog, and treat that dog to a really good walk a few times a day? If you were to spend a lot of money for home exercise equipment or hand weights, would you be sure to use the stuff? Would you enjoy a plan that involves the same type of exercise every day? Or would you prefer to mix it up with a variety of activities, to avoid boring yourself?

Are you a social person? If so, it might help you to exercise with a partner, or in group classes given at a sports club, senior center, or local YMCA. Would you like to hike or trek in the wilderness with a group of environmentally minded individuals, as in the Sierra Club? Would you go with a group to try cross-country or downhill skiing? Would any exercise program work best for you if it involved a family member or a friend who might also enjoy the diversion? Would it help you to keep moving if you simply bribe yourself? Do you need to draw up a legal contract with yourself and sign it? Will keeping written records help or discourage you?

You probably know what can help motivate you, and keep you motivated. Schedule physical activity to not conflict with your most important obligations to your job, family, and other facets of your life. Then find a way to work it into your life. Tailor the physical activity to your own fascinations and desires, but make it as regular as possible. Don't set your standards so high that you guarantee failure. Remember: *daily* exercise is best for reducing blood sugar.

GOLDEN RULES OF EXERCISE

Here are the two golden rules of physical activity or exercise:

I. Some exercise is better than none at all.
II. Regular exercise is even better.

The reason that *regular* physical activity is best doesn't just involve the calorie-burning benefits that last for several hours after you stop exercising. When you exercise regularly, after a few months your metabolism actually changes, and you burn more calories all day long.

If you become more physically active, you may also have less trouble changing your eating style. Certain hormones are released while exercising; these chemicals actually *decrease* rather than increase the appetite. Studies of laboratory rats reveal that rats eat more and fatten up if they are denied physical activity. The same is true of beef cattle fattened up on feedlots. While athletes in training frequently eat great quantities of food, they burn most of it off by exercising.

FEEL THE DIFFERENCE

When you begin your more physically active lifestyle, you should soon *feel* some improvement. Your blood sugar levels should begin to fall. With lower blood sugar, you should feel slightly more energetic, and a bit less tired and fatigued. In approximately a month and a half, your utilization of oxygen and your heart rate will improve.

From three to seven muscle-using sessions of twenty to thirty minutes per week may be a respectable goal. Sometimes, longer exercise sessions are recommended for promoting weight loss and increasing insulin sensitivity. The intensity and type of exercise or activity employed will vary, with each person encouraged to do what she can within safe limits to benefit themselves.

Most of us should start exercising gradually, and work our way up to longer sessions. Short, moderately strenuous daily exercise is preferable to exercise that is arduous, infrequent, and of high intensity. Remember that running guru and author Jim Fixx dropped dead of a heart attack while jogging. Don't overdo it. Moderate, regular activity is also helpful in losing weight. Ten years ago, 184 overweight Boston police officers went on low-calorie diets, and half also participated in an exercise program involving ninety-minute sessions three times a week. Results of the research published in *The American Journal of Clinical Nutrition* showed that the police officers who exercised not only lost more weight but kept it all off for years afterwards if they continued to exercise.

LIFESTYLE CHANGES

In the beginning, a little bit of physical activity is better than none. In small increments, try to step up the level of physical activity in your life. If fatigue is a problem, be sure to eat breakfast and other meals, drink plenty of water, get adequate sleep, and avoid sleeping pills. Getting a little sunlight in the morning, turning off the TV, and avoiding sitting in one spot for too long can increase your energy levels.

Studies have shown that great numbers of obese people don't move around much at all; if you are very overweight, simple activities such as vacuuming the house or dusting the furniture may be a good, productive way to begin exercising and shine up your home at the same time. If you sit in a cubicle at work, stand up every now and then, take a short walk down the hall, work out with some light hand weights, or do something during your breaks and lunch hour that involves moving your body. Using a cordless telephone allows you to pace back and forth when you talk. If it won't ruin your image, you might spurn the electric golf cart and walk, pulling your bag of clubs around the golf course.

Some individuals need to trick themselves to get started. Pulling the batteries out of the remote control for your television or CD player is a trick that works because it forces you to stand up and walk over to the set and switch channels by hand. Instead of bringing a heaping plate of snack food into the television area with you, force yourself to walk back into the kitchen every time you wish to grab a snack, and try to grab something nutritious. Or if you're at work, force yourself to walk around the block before or after allowing yourself to eat a doughnut. Start walking to the supermarket if that is possible, and make frequent trips. Unplug the automatic dishwasher, the electric egg beaters, and other appliances, and do some of the work by hand, the old-fashioned way. If you're overweight, you can begin to lower your blood sugar through modest increases in daily physical activity.

These days, almost all pregnant women are advised to exercise; limited exercise is even recommended for pregnant women with diabetes or gestational diabetes. Pregnant women with diabetes are often advised to begin an exercise program early, but exercise sessions are often kept short, limited to fifteen to thirty minutes to avoid depleting the supply of oxygen to the fetus. Exercises such as walking, bicycling, and swimming are frequently recommended, although some precautions apply in certain pregnancies. More on gestational diabetes may be found in chapter 12.

As you become more active, be sure to drink more water or other liquids to replace the body fluids that you lose during exercise. The human body is about 75 percent water, so we all need to drink a supply of it every day. Drinking more water helps your kidneys rapidly flush waste materials out of your system, a natural and healthy benefit to people with diabetes. Drinking plenty of water also prevents dehydration, which runs up the blood sugar. It's not a coincidence that almost every diet advises its practitioners to exercise and drink lots of water every day, because both are crucial factors not only in health, but also in weight loss.

As you become more physically active, you may choose to take on a program of exercise that is more structured, so that you can further improve your strength and help yourself.

BLOOD SUGAR CONTROL

For blood sugar control, Dr. Graham recommends taking a fifteen- to twenty-minute walk an hour or so after every meal, and also in the mornings. Mornings are a good time to walk because many people have high blood sugar then. Walking is a pleasurable activity that prevents blood sugar from rising as it normally does after a meal. Dr. Graham recommends checking blood sugar levels after the walk. This is particularly important for people on insulin, who need to coordinate the timing of their injections with meals and exercise.

Unless your blood sugar is unusually high, physical activity should be undertaken when your blood glucose is highest. This will help you manage and control your sugars. Blood sugar peaks and valleys vary from person to person. And unfortunately, most of us can't just drop everything we're doing and exercise at the ideal times. Any time you can exercise is the best time.

If your goal is weight loss, Dr. Graham recommends building up to longer sessions of up to an hour of continuous aerobic exercise. Sessions of this length are the most effective in any weight-loss program, she observes, because it takes thirty to forty-five minutes of aerobic activity before the body begins burning fat as a fuel.

AEROBIC EXERCISE

Aerobic exercise is an ideal form of exercise for people with diabetes because it directly lowers blood sugar. In addition, exercise physiologists often recommend an *anaerobic,* or weight training, type of exercise, and *muscle-stretching* exercises before and after workouts.

"Whenever I give a talk and mention aerobic exercise as the exercise of choice, the men in the audience always get a sort of glazed-over look," Dr. Graham has observed. "I think they have this image of wearing leotards and dancing to Jane Fonda tapes. The truth is *aerobic* simply means the exercise requires you to use more oxygen."

Aerobic exercise should be rhythmic and continuous. In addition to pumping more oxygen through the lungs, Dr. Graham defines aerobic exercise as any exercise which engages the major muscle groups such as the arms and legs, and increases the heart rate for at least twenty to thirty minutes, and which is performed at least three times a week. In people with adequate insulin, just thirty minutes of moderate aerobic exercise can cause up to a 20 to 25 percent decrease in blood glucose levels because the body becomes more sensitive to insulin and the muscles burn up glucose.

Always start slowly, and work your way up. Mild to moderate aerobic exercise is often preferred. The old rule of thumb is that if you can sing, you're moving too slowly, but if you can't talk, you're moving too fast. Gunnar Borg's Scale for Rate of Perceived Exertion is based on the idea that people can easily identify their own levels of exertion. Ideally, according to Borg's scale, aerobic exercise should be somewhere between exercise we perceive as fairly light and exercise we perceive as hard.

Moderate aerobic exercise can include activities such as walking, jogging, swimming, cycling, roller-skating, ice-skating, and cross-country skiing. All cause air to huff and puff through the lungs, and the heart to briskly pump oxygen to every part of the body. Moderate exercise is preferred to strenuous exercise for people with diabetes because moderate exercise burns the most fat and does not excessively deplete the glucose stored in the liver or muscles, as can long bouts of strenuous exercise. Water aerobics is a non-weight-bearing exercise that can build strength and aerobic capacity, because water supports the body and can provide plenty of resistance as well.

Walking briskly is a natural, weight-bearing aerobic exercise with many benefits. A study conducted in Australia followed a group of overweight postmenopausal women with and without Type 2 diabetes for three months. Each group was asked to walk an hour five times a week, without modifying their diets at all. The nondiabetic women didn't lose weight, but the women with diabetes lost 5.3 pounds, their HbA1c levels fell from 7.78 percent to 7.19 percent, their fasting glucose dropped from 167 to 148 mg/dl, and their cholesterol improved. One Los Angeles diabetes specialist states that taking a twenty-minute walk three times a week will add a year and a half of good life, while walking an hour a day adds three good years to the lifespans of people with diabetes.

Cross-country skiing is one of the best of all aerobic exercises. Folk dancing, square dancing, or ballroom dancing can be a sexy, social, and pleasurable aerobic activity. Choices abound. However, it may surprise you to learn that running a 50-yard dash is *not* considered aerobic exercise because it requires only a short, concentrated burst of energy. Aerobic exercise also does not include activities in which you move only once in a while, such as baseball, golf, or bowling; these are considered *anaerobic,* a word that means "without oxygen."

Do what you enjoy. Varying your workouts will help avoid injuries by stressing and toning different sets of muscles. Variety may keep you from becoming bored. The expenditure of enough energy to burn 150 calories is a good day's moderate activity, according to *The Commonsense Guide to Weight Loss*, by Barbara Hansen and Shauna Roberts. In less than an hour, you can burn 150 calories by gardening, washing windows, walking, dancing fast, washing and waxing your car, or wheeling yourself in a manual wheelchair. Playing basketball for fifteen to twenty minutes or pushing a baby stroller for a half hour accomplishes the same.

Being old—or even bedridden—should not prevent you from exercising. So-called armchair exercises can be a good form of exercise for people who are hospitalized or elderly, or who have limited mobility. Some of these exercises involve sitting in a chair and performing simple muscle-strengthening exercises and stretches. A few involve light weights or simple exercises that can be done to music. Senior citizens centers, hospitals, and some YMCAs offer group classes. Or videos may be purchased or rented for exercising at home.

In general, Dr. Graham says, the safest exercises for older people are those that support the body weight—aerobics, swimming, cycling, rowing, armchair exercises, and light strength training. More hazardous to older people are running programs, which put more than twice the stress on bones and joints as does walking. Proceed with caution when contemplating heavy weight lifting or isometric exercises, which can raise blood pressure. Exercises that require quick, rapid new movements are not recommended for most older people. Many of these recommendations also apply to people who are extremely overweight.

OTHER FORMS OF EXERCISE

In addition to aerobic exercise, your doctor or exercise physiologist may urge you to work other forms of exercise into your program of physical activity. Stretching and anaerobic exercises add safety and variety to your workouts.

Five or ten minutes of warmups and stretching before any exercise is recommended, particularly warmups that stretch the leg muscles. Stretching exercises are recommended because the nerve endings in the legs of people with diabetes can become dull, and you may not feel the normal sensation of pain in the ligaments that connect the muscles with the bones. Not noticing this pain can result in torn ligaments or broken bones in the foot. Purely for the sake of safety, it's important to stretch the Achilles tendon behind each ankle, as well as the calf and hamstring muscles. Stretching exercises increase flexibility, but are recommended only to the point of regular joint motion, *not* to the point of searing pain. After exercising, a few minutes of cool-down and stretching exercises are recommended by most doctors. Professional athletes do this to minimize injuries.

Weight training, also called resistance training or anaerobic exercise, is another form of exercise frequently recommended for people with diabetes because it can help to lower blood sugar. Proper techniques of lifting and breathing must be employed to minimize injury, or to compensate for any resulting rise in blood pressure. Weight training is *not* recommended if you have complications involving the eyes or kidneys, or if you have high blood pressure.

Among the benefits of weight training are improved muscle strength, increased lean body mass, increased bone density, and perhaps improved glycemic control. This form of exercise also strengthens bones and joints, and reduces the risks of injury in other types of exercise.

Weight-bearing exercise is particularly beneficial for women because it reduces the risk of *osteoporosis,* a disease in which calcium and other minerals are depleted from the skeleton, causing a brittleness of the bones. Women are at particular risk for osteoporosis because they lose certain hormones as they age, which contributes to bone loss. Diabetes accelerates bone loss in women, and to a lesser extent in men. Weight-bearing exercises can help minimize bone loss.

Weight-bearing exercise can be as simple as walking, which an estimated 40 million Americans claim as their exercise of choice. There's a lot to be said for this most natural form of exercise, including the fact that it's almost impossible to injure yourself while walking if you take sensible precautions with your feet. After all, our bodies were built to walk every day, searching for food and adventure. Walking briskly gets the heart and lungs working, but even a leisurely stroll at 3 miles an hour five days a week can raise HDL, or "good," cholesterol levels, according to a study of women walkers published in *The Journal of the American Medical Association*. Walking is inexpensive, and it may be done in your neighborhood or in any safe, scenic location, such as a park. Walking doesn't require special equipment or special training, and it can be done almost anywhere weather permits. As chapter 11 explains, daily foot care is important whether you walk or not.

The weather, the altitude, illness, injuries, smoking, drinking, taking medications, and other factors may require extra precautions, which should be explained to you by your doctor. If your doctor doesn't address these topics, ask about them.

SPORTS CLUBS

Sports clubs are great places to get a workout, and many have personal trainers on staff. If you prefer to exercise in the company of others, or if competition inspires you, sports clubs or exercise classes may be the way to go. Select a location that's fairly close to your home, so that it will be easy for you to get there.

Some commonsense precautions apply. The authors of *The Diabetes Sports and Exercise Book* recommend that you check out a club by asking specific questions about diabetes before you join. Will the club permit you to check your blood sugar between exercises, for instance, or do club officials become squeamish at the sight of blood? Will the club let you bring a small snack into the workout room to eat if your blood sugar gets low, or is there an ironclad rule against snacking? Before you join, meet with the club's personal trainer, if one is available, and find out if he or she knows anything about diabetes. Not every personal trainer knows the limits that should be placed on exercise for people with diabetes. If you determine that the club's trainer is ignorant about diabetes, and you still join the club, don't let that trainer put you into an exercise program not approved by your medical team. Don't do anything that sounds dangerous to you. For instance, don't do something as reckless and harmful to yourself as hanging upside down in gravity boots if you've got eye problems.

If the club checks out and the price is right, join it and take advantage of its services. In addition to a floor full of exotic-looking exercise machines, which you may enjoy like a kid discovering a new playground, many sports clubs also offer interesting exercise and dance classes at particular times.

Plain old community exercise classes are another alternative that will help you become more physically active, and they're less trouble than joining a sports club. Classes are offered by schools and community colleges, and through organizations such as the YMCA and YWCA. Senior citizens centers sometimes sponsor classes in such exotic disciplines as yoga, tai chi, aerobics, square dancing, swimming, and gymnastics. The YMCA offers good exercise classes for people with arthritis.

If you enjoy socializing while you exercise, many towns have mall-walking clubs, which offer group physical activity plus the distraction of high-speed window shopping in a cool, safe place. Mall-walking clubs typically meet early, before the mall opens its doors. They're a nice way for a business to share its facilities with the public. These clubs sometimes reward individuals who achieve certain personal milestones, such as walking their first thousand miles.

PRECAUTIONS TO TAKE

The benefits of exercise outweigh the risks in almost every person, but consult your doctor about any precautions you should take *before* you begin. Certain types of exercise are taboo with certain complications of diabetes, and with some medications. Of course, *never exercise when you are sick,* a topic covered in chapter 11. *Do not exercise if your blood glucose level exceeds 400 mg/dl at any time.*

If you exercise vigorously, don't forget to take a day off now and then to allow your body to recover. If you have laid off your exercise program for quite a while, your body will know it. After only a few weeks of bed rest and limited motion, you'll lose some of your muscle mass, oxygen-consuming capability, improved heart rate, and even a bit of calcium. You'll likely feel stiff and tired; you may be somewhat depressed. You may regain weight, and lose some control of your blood sugar. When you return to a more physically active lifestyle after being sick or bedridden, begin gradually, and slowly build back your strength over a month or two.

Although low blood sugar is rarely a problem for people with Type 2 diabetes, exercise can occasionally cause low blood sugar in people who take diabetes medications or insulin. In consultation with your doctor, you may reduce your insulin dosage prior to exercising. As a precaution, inject insulin in sites other than the muscles you'll be using for exercise—if you plan to jog, for instance, don't inject insulin into your legs. Carry a snack with you. Test your blood sugar. If your blood sugar is low, snack on quick-acting carbohydrates such as Life Savers, Skittles, or glucose tablets. Avoid low blood sugar by snacking before or during your exercise period, or by planning exercise during periods of peak blood glucose, such as early morning hours or sixty to ninety minutes after eating a meal. Do not drink alcohol right after exercising because it further lowers blood sugar. And if your exercise lasts all day, as in a wilderness hike, you'll need to eat something every hour.

If you take insulin or other diabetes medications, be on guard for immediate symptoms of low blood sugar such as shakiness, weakness, sweating, nervousness, dizziness, or hunger. Also watch for symptoms that can come on more slowly, such as irritability, confusion, drowsiness, headache, or poor coordination. Some symptoms of low blood sugar often accompany exercise—for instance, a quickly beating heart, or sweating. A quick blood sugar test will tell you for sure. Since some symptoms of low blood sugar are unique to the individual, keep your own history in mind. If your exercise or activity lasts longer than an hour, check your blood sugar *during* exercise.

People who exercise frequently are at a slightly higher risk for a rare condition called *postexercise, late-onset hypoglycemia,* or PEL. PEL may occur after long periods of exercise, or exercise of particularly high intensity. PEL is more likely to occur if you have been sedentary and suddenly begin an exercise program. PEL occurs because the exercise causes your body to become more sensitive to insulin, increasing your metabolism and causing sugar to be pulled out of storage in the liver and muscles. PEL can occur up to twenty-four hours after exercising. Extreme heat or cold weather can cause your body's insulin levels to fluctuate more than normal, so pay attention to how extremes in weather affect your blood sugars. If you exercise frequently, ask your doctor about PEL. Although PEL is rare, planning for it by testing your blood sugars after exercise will help you avoid it.

IT'S YOUR LIFE

Some people know the benefits of physical activity, but still find it difficult to work more exercise into their lives. It's hard to find time for exercise, some people say. They're too busy. They're too old. They're too sore.

They're too fat. They're too embarrassed. They're too afraid exercise might hurt. Consider the possibility that these may be unacceptable excuses.

The choice you have is between becoming more active or refusing to change.

It's difficult, but not impossible, to change your behavior. Make the decision to become more physically active. Look at it as a job, if that works for you. Every day, motivate yourself. Plan ahead, and exercise on time. Figure out tricks—and treats—that keep you motivated. Don't allow yourself too many lazy days off, and don't buy your own transparent excuses. One woman uses the "five minute rule." If she doesn't feel like exercising on a particular day, she forces herself to exercise for only five minutes. Afterward, if she still doesn't wish to exercise, she allows herself to stop.

To succeed, you must fit the physical activity to yourself. Start slowly, then build up to longer and more challenging sessions. Exercise at home, if that suits you. Join a club or exercise class if that motivates you. Be as active as possible as regularly as possible. Don't beat yourself up if you miss one session, or if you're sick or busy and happen to skip one day. Miss what time you absolutely must, then go back to living a more physically active lifestyle as soon as you can. If you must miss one session, immediately schedule another in its place. Set realistic goals that can be achieved.

Most important of all, permit yourself a moment or two *after* each exercise session to savor how well you really feel. Almost every human being feels better after exercising. The long-term benefits that you may not even notice should include greater physical strength, easier breathing, a better attitude toward yourself and your life, and perhaps even sounder sleep.

Along with these important lifestyle changes, medications may have a place in your self-management strategy. The next chapter looks at the medications that your doctor may prescribe in treating diabetes.

Chapter 9

DRUGS

A Look at Diabetes Pills and Insulin

~

IN ADDITION TO THE LIFESTYLE CHANGES DISCUSSED IN PREVIOUS CHAPTERS, SEVERAL drugs can be useful in the treatment of Type 2 diabetes. This chapter discusses the types of drugs that may be prescribed by your doctor, including diabetes pills and insulin. It explains what these drugs are, what benefits and side effects may occur, and how each drug may be employed in treating diabetes alone or in combination with other drugs. Some precautions regarding medications are also included.

At some point in your treatment, your doctor may suggest that you try one of the medications available to keep blood sugar at acceptable levels. These *oral hypoglycemic medications,* often called diabetes pills, are often used in tandem with diet and exercise to control blood sugar.

Diabetes pills may be prescribed when your treatment begins, at certain points along the way, or when lifestyle changes alone do not sufficiently lower blood sugar. Prescription drugs have side effects, so it's always useful to examine the risks and the rewards since this is what the doctor who treats your diabetes must do. Ask your doctor to explain the risks and benefits of diabetes pills, or of any medication he or she prescribes. Do understand that, despite some predictable side effects, no medicine when properly used in the treatment of diabetes will do as much harm to your body as prolonged levels of high blood sugar.

In more than three out of four cases of Type 2 diabetes, the body produces adequate insulin, but this insulin cannot be properly utilized by the body. In these cases, lifestyle changes may be enough to achieve blood sugar control. However, if you have the form of Type 2 diabetes sometimes called Type 2½, in which your body does not produce adequate insulin, you will not be able to control diabetes through lifestyle changes alone. Your doctor will prescribe either diabetes pills or insulin —in addition to lifestyle changes—and you will need medication to keep your blood sugars under control.

When you begin taking most diabetes pills or insulin, one unfortunate side effect is that you may gain weight. This is because blood sugar rushes into your cells. Even though you may have been eating a lot of food, your body has actually been in a fasting state, with excess glucose backed up in your bloodstream. Rather than being absorbed and oxidized for energy, this circulating sludge of glucose can't reach your body's cells. Medications help release your body from this state of artificial fasting and produce weight gain. Sugar will rush into your cells for several days after you begin taking these medications, and some of it will be stored as fat. One exception to this phenomenon among diabetes drugs is metformin, which normally causes weight loss. Acarbose, another new drug, does not promote weight gain.

Remember that diabetes medications work best within a coordinated program of lifestyle changes involving modifcations in eating style, efforts to reduce stress, and increased physical activity. This approach produces the quickest improvements in blood sugar.

DIABETES PILLS

Diabetes pills help people with diabetes utilize their own insulin more effectively. When diabetes pills are first prescribed, blood glucose levels frequently drop 15 to 20 percent.

Diabetes pills are normally not the first choice to get blood sugars under control. Most physicians prefer to first try lifestyle changes involving diet and exercise, attempting to bring blood sugars under control without medications. A few physicians do prescribe the oral agents first. After blood sugars are under control, they then add lifestyle changes to further bring down weight and blood sugar levels. Both strategies work. However, if your body manufactures adequate insulin, if you are vigorously pursuing lifestyle changes to lower your blood sugar, and you are making progress, you can ask your doctor for a little more time to get your blood sugar under control before you begin taking insulin or pills.

Diabetes pills are not a cure. Most of them work for a period of time, usually several years, then slowly lose their effectiveness. If the pills no longer provide adequate control of blood sugar, you are then started on insulin.

Side effects depend on the medication and the patient. Diabetes pills can cause unusually low blood sugar, or hypoglycemia. Hypoglycemia has occurred approximately 1 to 2 percent of the time with some medications in clinical trials. Other possible side effects from oral hypoglycemic agents include stomach upsets, appetite diminishment, rashes, and itching. Many of these side effects are normal when you begin taking a particular medication, but gradually disappear as your body learns to

USING DIABETES PILLS

The following precautions are recommended for people taking oral hypoglycemic agents, or diabetes pills:

- Take each pill before or with meals, as directed.
- Do not double up pills if you miss a dose.

tolerate the drug. Certain precautions are in order when combining diabetes pills with other medications.

NEW MEDICATIONS

Several experimental medications to treat diabetes are being developed by pharmaceutical companies, and a few will probably be approved for use by the U.S. Food and Drug Administration within the next few years. One new class of medications, the thiazolidinediones, marketed under the brand names Avandia, Actos, and Rezulin, work against insulin resistance in a new way. Another new medication, metformin (Glucophage) is from a class of drugs called biguanides, first developed in the 1920s but only recently approved for use in the United States. Precose and similar new medications such as Prandin and Glyset change the way your body digests food.

The new medicines act differently on the body than the older class of diabetes pills, called *sulfonylureas,* which are still prescribed to help control diabetes. The sulfonylureas stimulate the pancreas to produce more insulin, and they have helped millions of people with Type 2 diabetes keep their blood sugar levels under control for long periods of time.

The use of hypoglycemic agents is often suspended or replaced with insulin by your doctor during periods of great physical or mental stress, such as pregnancy, surgery, severe infections, or major trauma. Precautions are advised with these medications for elderly people of normal weight, who can have significant incidences of low blood sugar. Pregnant women or women with diabetes seeking to become pregnant should not take sulfonylurea medications because they increase the chance of complications during pregnancy. People allergic to other sulfa drugs rarely react to sulfonylureas, but just in case, you should tell your doctor if you have a particular sensitivity to sulfa drugs or any other medication.

According to a long-term study published by the University Group Diabetes Program in 1970, oral hypoglycemic agents can increase the chances of fatal heart complications, compared with control by diet or diet plus insulin.

Since most diabetes pills lose their effectiveness over time, new medications are increasingly being prescribed to supplement older ones. *Combination therapy* may extend the benefits of diabetes pills for a significant time.

Like any medications, diabetes pills should be taken as directed. This is almost always before meals or with meals. If you skip a pill, *never* try to make it up by taking two pills the next time. Simply go back on schedule by taking the prescribed dose at the next appropriate time.

If you're working to change your eating style, become more physically active, and reduce negative stress, you should not abandon those parts of your self-management program just because you've begun taking diabetes pills or insulin. Medications are not powerful enough to do the job by themselves, although they can be helpful. If your doctor has prescribed diabetes pills as a first step in a comprehensive strategy to help you control your blood sugar, you may be able to lower your recommended dose, or stop taking medications altogether, once you've achieved better control through lifestyle modifications.

AVAILABLE AGENTS

The following is a rundown of drugs that are prescribed for the treatment of diabetes, listed with the scientific name first and then brand names in parentheses. These listings summarize how particular medications work, and include normal dosage levels and the most common side effects. The newer medications metformin, acarbose, and troglitazone are listed first, followed by the sulfonylureas and the oldest effective drug for diabetes, insulin.

METFORMIN (GLUCOPHAGE)

This drug is a derivative of the French lilac, a traditional herbal remedy for diabetes in parts of Europe. Although new to the United States, metformin has been used in Europe and Canada for several years. Unlike the sulfonylureas, metformin does *not* stimulate the pancreas to produce more insulin. Instead, metformin reduces the liver's normal production of glucose, which is about a gram or two a day in most people. It also improves the body's response to insulin, increases the body's uptake of glucose, and reduces the absorption of sugars in the intestine. All of these effects usually result in lower blood sugar. Metformin can also reduce levels of triglycerides and other fats such as LDL, or "bad," cholesterol in the blood. Metformin works as an appetite suppressant in many people, so it is sometimes used as a diet pill by people who are not diabetic. One study showed an average weight loss of 8.4 pounds for people taking metformin. Another research study of metformin showed an average blood sugar decrease of 53 mg/dl.

Metformin cannot cause hypoglycemia, or low blood sugar, when taken alone. However, it may be used in combination with sulfonylurea drugs for additional drops in blood sugar levels. Metformin is not approved for use with insulin.

Metformin pills are white, in either 500 mg or 850 mg tablets. Typically, doses begin at one 500 mg tablet, and increase gradually to about 1,500 mg per day.

Side effects: Metformin may cause side effects in 10 to 30 percent of users, including loss of appetite, nausea, stomach upset, and diarrhea. These effects frequently subside over time (if not, the dose can be lowered). Approximately one-third of patients in clinical trials suffered side effects. Metformin can also cause a slight lowering of vitamin B-12 levels.

Precautions with metformin: Do *not* take metformin if you have a kidney problem, use alcohol excessively, or have severe congestive heart failure. The use of metformin with any of these can result in a serious and potentially fatal side effect, *lactic acidosis,* which results when body tissues don't get enough oxygen. Lactic acidosis can occur if metformin is given to people with plasma toxemia, or if it is given before having surgery or before receiving dye for imaging procedures.

ACARBOSE (PRECOSE)

This drug works in the small intestine to slow the breakdown of carbohydrates, particularly complex carbohydrates, thereby holding down the so-called *postprandial blood sugar rise* that normally occurs after eating. Technically an alpha-glucosidase inhibitor that does not act within the endocrine system, acarbose blocks the action of several enzymes such as glucomylase and sucrase, which help break down complex carbohydrates for absorption in the small intestine. Acarbose slows down the natural breakdown of starches, dextrins, maltose, and sucrose to absorbable monosaccharides. When taken alone it can lower blood sugar without the risk of hypoglycemia, hyperinsulinemia, lactic acidosis, or weight gain. Since acarbose evens out the blood sugar rise after eating, it is most effective in people who have their greatest problems with high glucose levels at that time.

The benefits of acarbose are proportional to carbohydrate intake—if you eat a lot of carbohydrates, acarbose has a greater effect. Acarbose is FDA approved as a combination therapy with a sulfonylurea. It has been used in combination with metformin and insulin.

Acarbose is taken just before meals, or with the first bite of each meal. Tablets are white to yellow-tinged in color. Use typically begins with 25 mg doses, or half a 50 mg tablet. Maximum dose is 50 to 100 mg per day, depending on the weight of the patient.

Side effects caused by undigested carbohydrates fermenting in the large intestine include abdominal pain, diarrhea, and flatulence, all of which can diminish after a month or two. However, some patients cannot tolerate these effects.

Precautions: Acarbose is *not* to be used with patients who have inflammatory bowel disease, colonic ulceration, or partial intestinal obstruction. There is a danger of low blood sugar reactions when acarbose is used in combination with sulfonylurea drugs.

REPAGLINIDE (PRANDIN)

Repaglinide is a chemical derivative of benzoic acid, which stimulates the beta cells in the pancreas to make more insulin, assisting glucose uptake. The first of a new group of diabetes drugs called the meglitinides, it acts quickly and dissipates quickly to suppress the glucose rise after a meal. It can be used as needed by people whose meals come at unpredictable times, and is taken before meals. Starting dose is 0.5 mg; maximum dose is 4 mg. Available in white 0.5-mg, yellow 1-mg, and red 2-mg tablets.

Side effects: Repaglinide can cause low blood glucose reactions and sinus or breathing problems. It carries a slightly higher risk of heart-related problems than some diabetes medications.

Precautions: Repaglinide can interact with other drugs, including troglitazone and drugs used to treat fungal or bacterial infections.

MIGITOL (GLYSET)

Migitol prevents the breakdown of carbohydrates in the intestines by inhibiting the action of certain enzymes, resulting in lower blood sugar levels after eating. Migitol may be employed as monotherapy or in combination with sulfonylureas. It can cause a slight weight loss or block or reduce a sulfonylurea-induced weight gain. Pills are white. Available in 25-mg, 50-mg, and 100-mg tablets. Starting dose is 25 mg; typical dose is 50 mg at mealtime.

Side effects include flatulence, diarrhea, and abdominal pain, and occasionally skin rash or lowered iron levels. Not recommended for patients with a renal dysfunction, inflammatory bowel disease, obstructions of the colon, or a predisposition to chronic intestinal diseases.

THE THIAZOLIDINEDIONES

The thiazolidinediones are a new group of drugs, working against insulin resistance by allowing cells to "open up" more normally and take in more glucose. They also decrease the production of glucose by the liver. The first of these was troglitazone (Rezulin), followed by rosiglitazone (Avandia), and pioglitazone (Actos). Troglitazone caused a stir when some patients reported liver damage, and has recently been pulled from the market. The two newest drugs from the so-called glitazone family, rosiglitazone (Avandia) and pioglitazone (Actos), have not been shown to damage the liver, but manufacturers are currently recommending periodic testing as a precaution.

ROSIGLITAZONE (AVANDIA)

Rosiglitazone acts by increasing insulin sensitivity, particularly in muscle and adipose tissue and in the liver. It reduces levels of free fatty acids and increases HDL and LDL cholesterol levels. It is taken once or twice daily, with or without meals, either in the morning or in the morning and the evening. Usual starting dose is 4 mg per day, which may be increased to 8 mg after three months if advised. Available in 2 mg, 4 mg, or 8 mg pink, orange, or brown tablets. Rosiglitazone may be used as monotherapy or in combination with metformin.

Side effects can include a slightly greater chance of upper respiratory tract infections, anemia, and edema. It can cause resumption of ovulation in women who have insulin resistance and have stopped ovulating; therefore birth-control measures are prudent.

Precautions: It is recommended to be used with caution in patients with edema, heart failure, or liver problems. Although it is believed to have no liver toxicity, periodic monitoring of liver enzymes is recommended by the manufacturer.

PIOGLITAZONE (ACTOS)

First manufactured in Japan, pioglitazone acts to lower blood sugar primarily by decreasing insulin resistance, which enhances the effects of circulating insulin in the liver and elsewhere in the body. It may be taken once a day, with or without meals. It achieves peak concentration within about two hours or a bit longer if food is ingested, and usually reduces triglyceride levels and increases HDL or "good" cholesterol levels in the blood. It can result in weight gain. It may be used in combination with sulfonylurea, metformin, and insulin. It is available in white to off-white 15 mg, 30 mg, and 45 mg tablets. Maximum dose is 45 mg per day as monotherapy, and 30 mg per day as part of combination therapy.

Side effects: Like other agents, it can increase the incidence of hypoglycemia. It causes an average 2 to 4 percent decline in hemoglobin and hemotocrit in blood. It can make birth-control pills less effective, indicating additional birth-control methods for women. It can cause increased possibility of mild to moderate edema, upper respiratory tract infections, headache, sinusitis, myalgia, and tooth disorders. Patients should immediately report unexplained nausea, vomiting, abdominal pain, fatigue, anorexia, or dark urine to their doctors.

Precautions: It should not be used in patients with liver disease or hepatic insufficiency. It should be used with caution in patients with edema.

SULFONYLUREA DRUGS

The sulfonylureas were discovered by accident during World War II. Researchers at work on sulfa antibiotics discovered that this particular class of sulfa drugs lowered blood sugar in the research subjects. This finding was soon applied to people with diabetes, who benefited from the side effect of lower blood sugar.

Sulfonylureas stimulate the pancreas to make more insulin, overcoming either a shortage of insulin or insulin resistance. At the end of their natural cycle, sulfonylurea drugs break down in the liver and are excreted. They can be safely taken for long periods of time, and often work effectively for years. Beginning these medications can produce a weight gain of 5 to 10 pounds.

Sulfonylurea compounds include the first-generation drugs tolbutamide, acetohexamide, tolazamide, and chlorpropamide, and the second-generation drugs glipizide, glyburide, and glimepiride. Several pharmaceutical companies make brand-name sulfonylurea drug products. The older compounds are available in generic form.

Sulfonylurea drugs are listed on the following pages, with the shortest-acting, first-generation agents listed first. Most sulfonylureas may be used in combination with insulin, but this increases the risk of low blood sugar.

Side effects of sulfonylureas can include occasional incidences of low blood sugar or hypoglycemia, headache, nausea, flushing of face, dizziness, diarrhea, skin rashes, and increased urination. The second-generation sulfonylureas do not have the side effect of increased urination, but they are a bit more likely to cause low blood sugar because their active ingredients are more concentrated and therefore more effective. If you are just beginning to take diabetes pills, watch out for symptoms of low blood sugar such as sweating, shakiness, dizziness, difficult or slurred speech, hunger, blurry vision, nausea, mental confusion, or irritability. Low blood sugar may occur after or during strenuous exercise, or when you skip a meal. If you suspect low blood sugar at any time, test yourself. If your blood sugar is low, simply eat a snack and you'll be fine.

FIRST GENERATION

Tolbutamide (Orinase)—A short-acting medication that starts working in an hour, and is gone within six to twelve hours. The only short-acting diabetes medication, tolbutamide comes in 250 and 500 mg white tablets, usually taken two to three times per day. Doses range between 500 and 3,000 mg per day.

Acetohexamide (Dymelor)—This medication starts working within an hour, and remains in the body for ten to fourteen hours. Available in 150 and 500 mg tablets, it is usually taken one to two times per day. Maximum dose is 1.5 grams, or 1,500 mg, per day.

Special precautions: Not to be used with patients having kidney problems.

Tolazamide (Tolinase)—This medication is prescribed for people who absorb their food very slowly; its onset is from four to six hours after ingestion. Tolazamide comes in 100, 250, and 500 mg white tablets and is usually taken one to two times per day. Maximum recommended dose is 1 gram, or 1,000 mg, per day.

Chlorpropamide (Diabinese)—Action starts in about an hour, but it stays in the body about seventy-two hours, making it the longest lasting of the sulfonylureas. It is available in 100 and 250 mg blue tablets. The maximum recommended dose is 500 mg per day, and it is taken once per day.

Side effects include a diuretic effect causing frequent urination, vascular problems with symptoms such as headache or flushing of the face, and an Antabuse-type reaction when taken with alcohol, causing a red, flushed face.

Precautions: Chlorpropamide is not recommended for anyone with kidney problems, or for elderly people.

SECOND GENERATION

Glipizide (Glucotrol, Glucotrol XL)—Action begins an hour after ingestion, and it remains in the body for twelve to sixteen hours. Glipizide is to be taken on an empty stomach, about thirty minutes before a meal. This drug can even out blood sugar levels during the day. It can be used effectively in combination with insulin—one study found that subjects taking glipizide with insulin used only 48 units of insulin, compared to 77 units of insulin taken by subjects using insulin alone. Glipizide is available in 5 mg and 10 mg white tablets. It is taken one to two times per day. A maximum dose for most forms of glipizide is 40 mg per day, but for Glucotrol XL, the maximum is 20 mg per day.

Precautions: This drug is not normally prescribed for elderly patients.

Glyburide (Micronase, Diabeta, Glynase Prestabs)—An intermediate-acting oral agent, glyburide's effects begin in about an hour and a half, and it remains in the body for a maximum of twenty-four hours. It is available in 1.25 mg, 1.5 mg, 2.5 mg, 3 mg, 5 mg, and 6 mg tablets. The smallest available doses for each brand are white tablets; larger doses have pink, blue, or light green tablets, depending on the manufacturer. It is taken one to two times per day. The maximum dose is 20 mg per day.

Precaution: Caution is urged for the use of this medication by elderly people.

Glimepiride (Amaryl)—This may be taken once a day, to even out blood sugar over the course of a day. It is taken one time with breakfast or the first main meal of the day, usually beginning with 1 to

2 mg doses. Usual maintenance dose is 1 to 4 mg: it is available as 1 mg pink tablets, 2 mg green tablets, and 4 mg blue tablets. The maximum dose is 8 mg per day.

GENERIC DRUGS

Your medical doctor may specify on a prescription that a brand name rather than a generic drug is to be dispensed. However, there's now a trend toward the use of less expensive generic drugs whenever they are available. Many health-care providers now encourage the use of generic drugs, sometimes by offering the incentive of a lower co-payment if you choose a drug in its generic form. Using generic drugs is not quite the same as buying the house brand at the supermarket, although there are similarities. Pharmacists can be helpful in explaining the differences between brand name and generic drugs. Since profit margins are actually higher on generic drugs, if your pharmacist advises you to choose a brand name, strongly consider taking that advice.

Any pill is composed of two elements. The first is the amount of active ingredient by weight. This is always the same in both brand name and generic drugs. The second, much larger portion is what's in the rest of the pill—the so-called excipients, which can include coloring agents, binders, and fillers. Excipients can make a subtle difference in how much of the active ingredient your body will absorb, and how quickly the active element will move into your bloodstream. If you are sensitive to particular medicines, this difference can be significant.

The formulations of generic drugs may vary from generic brand to generic brand. Not all generic drugs are exactly the same, although all contain the same amount of the active ingredient, which is why you purchase a particular drug in the first place.

If you switch from a brand name to a generic form of a drug, or vice versa, pay attention to the drug's effects on your body and let your doctor know if you experience a problem. The dose you take may need to be adjusted.

SECONDARY FAILURE

For approximately one in five people with Type 2 diabetes, treatment with oral sulfonylureas may be effective for longer than ten years, and occasionally for as long as twenty or twenty-five years. However, the results are typically less long lived. The average time that these medications work to their full effect is between five and seven years, at which point their effectiveness dims.

For some reason that doctors still don't understand, diabetes pills do not work at all on approximately one-third of the people who try them. The reasons for these so-called *primary failures* are not clear, but they happen in the beginning and over time. Diabetes pills continue to lose their effectiveness in another 5 to 10 percent of the people taking them each year, a phenomenon called *secondary failure.*

These failures are sometimes temporary, caused by illness, stress, or an infection—doses of insulin may be prescribed to get you over the physical or mental stress that instigated the failure, and you may start taking the diabetes pills again. Secondary failures may also be permanent; researchers speculate that they may occur because the body becomes more resistant to its own insulin.

When one drug doesn't work or stops working, one possibility is to switch to another type of diabetes pill. This can work. For instance, your doctor might begin with a sulfonylurea, then switch you to metformin. Another physician facing the same situation might choose to combine medications, prescribing a sulfonylurea and metformin, or a sulfonylurea and acarbose, but in lower doses for each. Such switches or combination therapy can often extend the period of effectiveness of drug treatments.

When medications begin to lose effectiveness, some physicians prefer a period of time with the diabetes pills, plus insulin injections in the evening, rather than switching to multiple insulin injections immediately and abandoning the diabetes pills. This can be an effective halfway step because lower doses of insulin are required when diabetes pills are taken. Another strategy is to begin insulin injections when the diabetes pills fail.

On the horizon are a few promising new oral hypoglycemic agents, currently in clinical trials throughout the world. Some, including newer formulations of sulfonylurea drugs, may assure a more consistent level of blood glucose all day long on just one dose per day.

INSULIN

An everyday necessity for people with Type 1 diabetes, supplemental insulin is used more sparingly in the treatment of Type 2 diabetes. Insulin often begins after hypoglycemic medications have lost their ability to control blood sugar. A good indicator of when to add insulin to your therapy is if your HbA1c level stays over 8 on a program involving diet, regular exercise, and diabetes medications. For people whose insulin production is below normal, supplemental insulin may be recommended right away.

While the idea of giving yourself shots may be frightening, understand that insulin will always help you control blood sugar. Better control can help prevent complications. When medical doctors are given the choice between good blood sugar control with supplemental insulin or poor control without it, the choice is always good control with insulin because the benefits far outweigh the risks to the patient's health.

It has been estimated that 20 to 50 percent of people with Type 2 diabetes may one day need insulin because the production of insulin by the pancreas slowly decreases in all people as they age.

Fortunately, insulin is one of the least expensive drugs on the market, and one of the most useful to people who require it. Insulin keeps people alive, and in some respects it's as close as scientists have come to discovering a miracle drug for diabetes. Before the discovery of insulin, people with Type 2 diabetes who no longer produced adequate insulin could expect to live for several years, but to function poorly and suffer many serious complications, such as blindness and gangrene. This is no longer the case.

The discovery of insulin in 1921 by Canadian researchers Frederick Banting and Charles Best was a major breakthrough in twentieth-century medicine. By injecting a primitive form of insulin into a dog whose pancreas had been removed, Banting and Best were able to keep the animal alive even though it produced no insulin of its own. This discovery extended many human lives.

The first insulin was made crudely, by grinding up the pancreases of pigs or cows; early users sometimes experienced side effects and autoimmune reactions caused by impurities. Today, human insulin is grown in huge lots, almost like biological farms. Commercial insulin derived from human insulin has been genetically engineered to clone itself on simple living organisms such as yeast or bacteria, resulting in a pure product. Although pork insulin is still manufactured, beef-pork insulin was phased out in 1999, despite protests from some users who felt this later-peaking insulin gave them superior control. Eli Lilly and Novo Nordisk are the only two companies in the United States that manufacture insulin.

TWO STRENGTHS OF INSULIN

The two strengths of insulin are U-100 and U-500. U-100 means that there are 100 units of insulin per cubic centimeter. Almost everyone uses U-100 insulin; U-500 is only used for research purposes. In other countries, insulin is manufactured in various strengths, but most of them have begun to adopt U.S. insulin standards.

Insulin is available in three types, all of which have different rates of absorption, different peaks, and different rates of time that they remain in the bloodstream. The three types are regular, or rapid-acting, insulin; intermediate-acting insulin; and long-acting insulin. All three are also known by other names.

TYPES OF INSULIN

Long-acting, or Ultralente, insulin begins working from four to eight hours after injection, peaks twelve to eighteen hours after injection, and remains in the body for twenty-eight hours or more.

Intermediate-acting, or *NPH,* or *Lente* insulin begins working from one to three hours after injection, peaks in six to twelve hours, and may not dissipate for eighteen hours.

Rapid-acting, or regular, insulin begins working about half an hour after injection, peaks in two to four hours, and dissipates after six to eight hours.

Lispro (Humalog). Besides the three major types of insulin, a new type called Lispro insulin was recently approved for commercial use by the U.S. Food and Drug Administration. Lispro is an insulin analog, sold under the brand name Humalog. The first so-called designer insulin, Lispro works and dissipates quickly; it is advantageous to take it just before eating if insulin is needed at mealtime. Lispro insulin can be taken only five or ten minutes before a meal (compared to at least thirty minutes for regular insulin). Lispro peaks about the same time that your blood sugar does after eating, but is gone within a few hours. Other new insulin analogs with different characteristics are in development.

Since none of these types of insulin is ideal, premixed combinations of regular- and intermediate-acting insulin are sold in the United States. These include 70/30 and 50/50 mixtures. Your physician may recommend that you take one of these combinations before meals, to provide fast insulin for the first-phase insulin response after eating (this response is often impaired in people with Type 2 diabetes), and to help with long-term effects. Premixed insulins are usually best for people with stable insulin needs.

Other mixtures such as 60/40 and 90/10 are sold in Europe. For this reason, take a supply of insulin with you when traveling, and find out beforehand what's available in the countries that you will be visiting.

YOUR INSULIN DOSE

To a great extent, your exact dosage of insulin will be worked out as you go along. In the beginning, your physician will recommend a strategy for controlling your blood sugar by using insulin. Blood glucose testing will tell you and your doctor how your body is using the insulin that you are taking. Frequent tests will identify adjustments that should be made, to compensate for changes in your blood sugar levels. Once a dosage and a schedule are established, use the same dose in the same amount, every day at the same time, unless your doctor makes another recommendation.

You should be in frequent contact with your health-care team when you begin taking insulin because finding the right dose can involve some trial and error. For instance, you may need more insulin if you smoke. A study of smokers with diabetes, conducted at University Hospital in Copenhagen, found that they required 15 to 20 percent more insulin than did nonsmokers with diabetes.

A schedule of injections that follows the natural pattern of your blood sugar fluctuations can be found; when you follow this pattern you will probably feel better immediately. With the exception of Lispro, insulin is typically taken thirty minutes before a meal because it has a delayed reaction of thirty to forty-five minutes before it begins working.

Your insulin dose will be given at specified times of day. Your life, especially your meal and snack times, will have to become more predictable when you take insulin. Watching the effects of insulin will allow you to space out your doses to accommodate your body's needs.

Remember that whether or not you use insulin, your eating schedule, exercise schedule, and stress level also affect your blood sugar. Insulin helps even out blood sugar fluctuations, but it can cause low blood sugar. Your blood sugar goals should be determined by you and your health-care team, based on your health history and age. Make sure that your doctor tells you what test results should prompt you to call.

TAKING INSULIN

At the present time, insulin must be introduced into the body through the skin. You may inject insulin yourself, or ask another person such as your spouse or a private nurse to do it. Most people find it convenient to inject themselves. Several devices are on the market to allow even people with a needle phobia to take insulin. Pharmaceutical companies are also working to develop an insulin that can be taken in pill form, but their attempts have been unsuccessful because the acids in the stomach and intestines break down the insulin before it can move into the bloodstream, where it does its work.

Insulin may be injected with a *syringe,* an automatic injection device called a *syringe autoinjector,* a type of air gun called a *hydrospray injector,* or a device called an *insulin infusion pump.* If you take insulin, you will need to learn how to measure a proper dose for yourself, and how to inject it underneath your skin, into your fatty tissue. Sites to inject insulin include the abdomen (often a preferred site), under the skin in the back of the arms, the upper buttocks, and the front of the legs. As a general rule, the higher up on the body that you inject insulin, the faster the insulin will peak. Recognizing these differences by tracking glucose levels when you begin is a better strategy than random selection of sites. Work with your medical doctor or your diabetes educator when you begin site rotation to find which sites give you best control at different times of the day. For some people, a good strategy is to take the breakfast and lunch shots in the arms so the insulin takes effect quickly, and to take dinner and bedtime shots in the thighs and buttocks where the usually slower absorption helps carry them through the night a bit better.

In the hospital, insulin may be administered intravenously (directly into the vein) through an IV, which is the fastest way to receive it. Insulin is sometimes injected by syringe into the muscle, where it acts more quickly than when it is injected subcutaneously (under the skin).

Insulin needles are short and slender, and cause little pain. Syringes cost about twenty cents apiece, and are the least expensive way to administer insulin. For another thirty to forty dollars, injection devices can make it easier to get insulin into your system if you are squeamish about needles. Insulin "pens," sold under names such as Accupen and NovoPen, use insulin cartridges. Autoinjection devices, sold under brand names such as Autojector, Inject-Ease, Injectomatic, and Monoject, work when you push a plunger button to get the needle, or the needle and the insulin, under your skin.

Jet injectors, which cost between $600 and $1,400 and are sold under brand names such as Medi-Jector II, Tender Touch, Preci-Jet 50, and Vitaject II, actually blow the insulin through the skin, with the depth of penetration adjustable by a nozzle in the unit that must be kept scrupulously clean.

The newest and most sophisticated device is the insulin infusion pump. Manufactured by companies such as MiniMed and Disatronic, pumps presently cost $4,500 to $5,000. In short intervals, or pulses, throughout the day, they provide insulin through a small needle or catheter placed under the skin into the subcutaneous tissue, mimicking the natural production of insulin by the pancreas. Insulin pumps are not automatic because they cannot regulate the flow of insulin to compensate for changes in blood sugar; this must be done manually based on blood sugar test results. Los Angeles physician Paul Sogol, M.D., reports that MiniMed has developed a special needle that, when inserted subcutaneously, acts as a continuous glucose sensor, and that one day will hopefully act with the insulin pump to regulate the flow of insulin based on blood sugar levels.

Pumps must be cleaned and loaded carefully, but they can provide tight control of blood sugars. For a detailed explanation of insulin pumps, see a book such as *Pumping Insulin,* by John Walsh and Ruth Roberts.

INSULIN INJECTIONS

When using a syringe at home to inject insulin subcutaneously, as most people do, certain steps must be followed. These include properly measuring the amount of insulin and maintaining a clean, sanitary environment.

Syringes are disposable; the labels say to dispose of them immediately after use. However, some people reuse their own syringes as many as four times because there is little danger of spreading disease when only one person uses the syringe. If this is done, the syringe should be cleaned and capped after use. When the needle has difficulty penetrating the skin, or when the injection begins to hurt, it's time for a new syringe.

People who have a fear of needles sometimes find that they can overcome their phobia by not using rubbing alcohol to rub down their arm because the smell of alcohol frequently triggers the fear. Special equipment is available to help people who are blind or partially sighted get the right dose of insulin into the syringe, and to read the syringe itself prior to injection. Classes on how to inject insulin and care for

INJECTING INSULIN

The basic steps for injecting insulin with a syringe are:

- Roll the insulin bottle between your palms, upside down and sideways.
- Clean the top of the bottle with alcohol on a cotton swab or wipe (clean the tops of both bottles if you are mixing insulins).
- Wash your hands.
- Draw air into the syringe by pulling out the plunger.
- Using the syringe, push air down the top of the bottle.
- Turning the bottle upside down, pull insulin into the syringe, avoiding air bubbles, to your dose level.
- Clean the injection site with an alcohol swab.
- Pinch your skin with your fingers, then insert the needle into the skin.
- Inject the insulin.
- Release the skin, pull out the needle, and lay it aside.
- Gently press the injection site to stop bleeding if it occurs—don't rub this area.

yourself when having a sight impairment are offered through organizations such as the Braille Institute and the American Foundation for the Blind; their telephone numbers and addresses are listed in the "Other Resources" appendix at the back of this book.

If you inject insulin, regularly rotate your injections around various parts of the body. A regular rotation of injection locations will prevent *hypertrophy,* a swollen or enlarged patch of skin that results when insulin is injected into the same location too many times. The doctor who treats your diabetes should check for hypertrophy when he examines you, even though this condition is becoming rare because of the purity of commercial insulin.

If you are using more than one type of insulin, diabetes educators Diana and Richard Guthrie suggest in *The Diabetes Sourcebook* that insulin bottles be color-coded or marked so that you can easily identify which one to inject at a particular time. Tape or rubber bands can also be used. The two U.S. insulin manufacturers are working with the FDA on a system of tactile identification of insulin vials, using bars or markings in braille. A standardized tactile marking system will benefit blind or partially sighted people who must use more than one type of insulin.

OBTAINING INSULIN

You don't need a doctor's prescription to purchase insulin in the United States. An exception to this is the new insulin, Lispro, which requires a prescription. The original insulin regulations were instituted so that people with diabetes could get insulin in an emergency. Some states do regulate the purchase of syringes.

When you are traveling, always carry either your doctor's prescription or the name of your insulin written on a piece of paper. Tearing off the top of your insulin box and putting it into your wallet or purse will usually do the trick.

Insulin bottles are marked with an expiration date, just like milk and other perishable items. Manufacturers won't guarantee their potency past this date. Insulin must be stored properly—kept in the refrigerator, but not frozen. If possible, keep an extra bottle on hand of the insulin that you are using.

Bottles in current use may be kept at room temperature, but avoid temperature extremes. Don't store insulin in direct sunlight, near heaters, or near ice. Insulin stored at room temperature begins to lose its potency after about a month; if that happens, the insulin should be tossed out even if some remains in the bottle.

Disposal of insulin syringes is a nuisance. Used syringes should be placed in a sturdy container such as a coffee can with a lid, then taped securely shut. Add bleach to the container when full, and dispose according to local regulations. Special disposal pouches are also sold. If you don't know what the regulations are regarding needle disposal, ask your city sanitation department's public relations office. Don't just toss used needles into the trash—they can be picked up by curious children, or by drug addicts. An improperly discarded syringe can spread disease.

Insulin is a wonder drug, one that can keep you alive and in better health when properly used. Remember that the basic idea is to coordinate the use of insulin with the rise and fall of glucose within your body. Striving for an insulin peak at about the same time as your blood sugars are expected to peak allows you maximum blood sugar control.

In addition to low blood sugar, side effects of insulin can include high blood pressure and headaches. Even if you're completely controlling your diabetes through diet and exercise, you still have diabetes; you may need life-saving insulin if you have a health problem and are hospitalized.

COORDINATING MEDICATIONS

Always tell the doctor who treats your diabetes what other medications you are taking because those medications can interact with diabetes drugs. Most diabetes pills should be cautiously taken with other drugs that affect blood sugar control, such as diuretics and beta blockers. These medications are often prescribed for high blood pressure, which frequently needs to be controlled in people with diabetes. Pain relievers such as the non-steroidal anti-inflammatory drugs (NSAIDs) and many other highly protein-bound medications can lower blood sugar. If you are treated by a specialist for another medical problem, *always* tell that doctor which diabetes medications you take. A specialist will not automatically receive this information. You can prepare a list of the medications that you take and hand it to any doctor.

In addition to the problem of drug interactions, drugstores occasionally make mistakes on prescriptions, and hospitals sometimes make mistakes in administering drugs. Errors can include errors in dosages or frequency in administering medications. Occasionally a pharmacist misreads a prescription—mistaking Humalog, a rapidly acting insulin, with Humulin, another type of insulin, or a prostate treatment drug such as Proscar for a diabetes treatment drug such as Precose. Do what you can to make sure you're taking the correct medicine in the correct amounts.

The doctor who treats your diabetes will help you assess the risks and benefits of medications in your treatment. If you experience a side effect that you don't understand, call your doctor and ask about it.

"Diabetes is a very complex thing because other conditions that you have can affect it," observed the owner of a construction company who has diabetes. "You can have certain symptoms, and not be sure if they're coming from the diabetes or from other things. The trick is to sort all the symptoms out and to figure out what it is that affects how you feel. You have to really educate yourself and find out about it to know for sure."

DRUGS THAT RAISE BLOOD SUGAR

While insulin and hypoglycemic agents lower blood sugar, other medications can raise blood sugar levels, throwing off glycemic control. The following drugs can raise blood sugar, and should be reported to the doctor who treats your diabetes:

- diuretics including thiazides
- corticosteroids
- phenothiazines
- thyroid products
- estrogen
- oral contraceptives
- phenytoin
- nicotinic acid
- sympathomimetics
- isoniazid

Oral hypoglycemic agents and insulin have an established place in the treatment of diabetes, but neither is a reason to give up on the lifestyle changes that are proven to help control blood sugar. Always take medication as directed, and report any problems to your doctor. If you need insulin, work with your doctor to arrive at the optimum dose for you. Combinations of diabetes pills, or pills and insulin, are sometimes useful in the treatment of diabetes. And, of course, test your blood sugar levels as directed by your health-care team. Home glucose testing will help you, as may the commonly performed medical tests explained in the next chapter.

Chapter 10

LAB TESTS

Laboratory Tests You May Receive and
Why They're Important

~

LABORATORY TESTS WILL BE GIVEN TO YOU BY THE DOCTOR WHO IS TREATING YOUR diabetes. Knowing when to expect these tests and how to interpret the results will improve your self-management. Understanding what each test actually measures and records may help you to focus on the results that are most significant, and stop you from worrying about numbers that don't matter much. All of this can help to empower you.

From time to time, you'll visit the doctor who is treating your diabetes. Your doctor will look at your eyes because this is the one opening in the human body in which a medical professional can actually see the condition of your blood vessels. Your doctor will check your reflexes, look at your feet, and do a general examination covering the important points listed in chapter 3. The doctor should ask to see your own blood sugar test records, and should arrange for you to receive laboratory tests to check your physical condition.

Interpreting the results of laboratory tests is an important part of your doctor's job. Understanding these results can be useful to you. Testing provides information on how well you are controlling your blood sugar and the levels of fat in your blood. Tests help your physician assess the condition of important parts of your body such as your vascular system and kidneys. You will probably receive several tests early on to establish a *baseline* against which subsequent test results may be measured.

The most common medical tests given to people with diabetes include blood pressure, glycosylated hemoglobin, a lipid profile that measures levels of fats such as cholesterol, and detection of protein in the urine. All of these tests should be given regularly to people with diabetes, and the results carefully evaluated. Specialized urine tests that can detect a loss of kidney function are useful in the treatment of kidney disease. Other tests that may be given are the oral glucose tolerance test and the fructosamine assay, typically given to pregnant women.

To your doctor, test results are merely pieces of information used to monitor and treat your disease. Your doctor may not share test results with you as a matter of course. If you're worried, or if you simply want to know, ask for the results of any test. While most of the tests listed in this chapter are given in your doctor's office, in some instances you may be required to do additional testing in your home. Some insurance plans reimburse for blood pressure monitors, which are used to check blood pressure at home. The most accurate home blood pressure test in current use is the mercury sphygmomanometer, which is typically seen in doctors' offices and is the most difficult to use at home. Aneroid monitors display results on a dial, but need to be recalibrated once a year or so, a service that is usually inexpensive. Home cholesterol tests are available, as are home tests for urinary tract infections. HbA1c tests and fructosamine meters for home use are also available, and are particularly valuable because they give longer-term reads on glucose control than those given by finger-stick tests.

You may choose to keep your own records, or copies of all of your medical tests. Keeping your own personal *medical records file* may be quite useful, especially if you must change doctors or health plans. In your logbook or file, write down all your test results, including the name of the doctor who performed the test and the date given. Or you may request computer printouts or photocopies of test results and file them. A medical records file provides a central reference point for information on your physical health. Having this data in one location, such as a loose-leaf notebook or a file in your personal computer, allows you to compare results from doctor visit to doctor visit, or simply to pat yourself on the back when the numbers improve. A few people even make graphs with this information, so that they can see their progress. Keeping your own medical file allows you to have information on hand if you need it in an emergency, or if you visit another specialist. You may wish to note any comments that your doctor makes to you in interpreting your test results, or in prescribing medication.

As a medical consumer and as a patient who is attempting to form a partnership with his or her physician, you always have the *right* to know your test results. This is true whether tests are given in a doctor's office, a laboratory, or a hospital. If you wish to know the results of tests that you are given, *ask*. Some doctors make it a practice to routinely share this information; others limit discussions about numbers and scientific tests because such information confuses some patients. Many people are bewildered or frightened by the medical system, and have trouble remembering all the things that they are told.

If you believe your test results are higher than they should be, and your doctor doesn't mention it or make suggestions to bring the numbers down, ask him or her to take a minute to explain the results. Ask if there's something you can do to improve your results, or whether it's safe to ignore them. Remember, if you're a full partner in your treatment, you must spell out your concerns and take on some responsibility. In this partnership, it's your job to point out to your doctor things that he or she may not have noticed.

BLOOD PRESSURE

Your blood pressure should be checked every time you visit a doctor. A blood pressure test is a simple, noninvasive method of testing the pressure inside your blood vessels, through which blood continually circulates, driven by the beating of your heart. High blood pressure may indicate that your blood vessels are constricted because of deposits of plaque, cholesterol, or other substances clinging to blood vessel walls. High blood pressure is called *hypertension*. You and your doctor should take steps to lower your blood pressure if tests show that it's too high.

The Hypertension Optimal Treatment Study, completed in 1998, found that lowering the diastolic blood pressure to 83 mmHG rather than 90 could reduce the incidence of heart attacks by more than one third in people with diabetes and that reducing this to 80 could cut risks in half. However, these are admittedly difficult numbers to obtain.

Normal blood pressure is 120/80 mmHG; numbers a few points different than these are of little concern. The first stirrings of high blood pressure are readings that are higher than 140 mmHG before the written slash, or higher than 80 mmHG after the written slash. Blood pressure above these numbers is dangerous and should be treated. Blood pressure in the range of 200/140 is considered extremely high. High blood pressure may be treated with medications or changes in diet, including lowering your salt intake.

Table 10.1 Blood Pressure

Normal	120/80 mmHG
High	140/80 mmHG
Extremely High	200/140 mmHG

HEMOGLOBIN A1C TEST

The *Hemoglobin A1C* or *glycosylated hemoglobin* tests are the gold standard of all diabetes testing. The two tests are almost identical, but because they examine a different subset of proteins in the red blood cells, their results may be expressed differently. At least two of these tests per year are recommended by the American Diabetes Association.

Given in your doctor's office or a laboratory, the glycosylated hemoglobin test gives your doctor a precise reading of your average blood sugar levels over the past few months. Knowing your average blood sugar levels shows you how successful you've been in your overall efforts to control blood sugar because your own test results will be higher or lower than your average. This test is sometimes used to diagnose diabetes.

The glycosylated hemoglobin test calculates your average blood sugar levels over the previous eight to twelve weeks, which is about the life of a red blood cell. Red blood cells are continually wearing out and being replaced in the human body. Hemoglobin is the red iron-rich protein in red blood cells, which carry oxygen. Over time, hemoglobin attracts glucose in proportion to the amount of glucose present in the blood.

Normal glycosylated hemoglobin levels range from 2 to 6 percent, depending on the test and the laboratory interpreting the results. The test results are equivalent to average blood sugar levels.

Many doctors set goals for their patients that are 1 percent higher than normal. Readings above eight or nine are considered serious.

The average reading for a person with diabetes in the United States is a 10, which is much too high. The United Kingdom Prospective Diabetes Study, or UKPDS trial, established a 7.1 percent HbA1c as ideal for people with Type 2 diabetes. Researchers in that trial noted that each percentage point reduction in this test level led to a 35 percent reduction in complications. An out-of-control person with diabetes may have glycosylated hemoglobin levels of 15 to 17 percent, which indicates that blood sugars have remained much too high over the past several weeks.

Note, however, that the glycosylated hemoglobin test is *not* a substitute for blood glucose testing at home. This is because glycosylated hemoglobin results in the average range don't always mean that you've consistently kept your blood sugars in perfect control. Blood sugars may have bounced up and down, averaging out to a normal reading on the test even though control has actually been poor. Anemia can skew the results. However, if you've made a serious effort to control your blood sugars, the results should be accurate and in line with those you recorded at home.

Ask for the equivalent blood sugar level for your test results. If your own results don't jibe with the doctor's results, it's possible that you may not be testing properly. Make an appointment with your doctor or nurse educator to check your technique. Check the accuracy of your blood glucose meter. A problem with your technique or your meter is more likely than a bad reading of your test, although laboratory misinterpretation of test results occasionally happens.

The glycosylated hemoglobin and Hemoglobin A1C tests are objective. The results will be accurate even if your blood sugar level is high or low on the day that you take it. This test yields a number that is useful to patient and doctor because it evaluates blood sugar control over a period of time. Many doctors say that patients should know this test result number as well as they know their cholesterol level, because it is extremely important. These tests should be standardized into one test to be given to all people with diabetes, but until this happens, comparing numbers from one type of test to another will remain difficult and confusing. One medical company is working on a noninvasive form of this test that would not draw blood, but would take measurements through a beam of light directed into the retina, a concept still in the preliminary stages.

Table 10.2	Glycosylated Hemoglobin Levels
3.5-6.2%	Normal
3.5-7.5%	Good Control
7.7-8.9%	Fair Control
9.0% and up	Poor Control

COMPARING HEMOGLOBIN A1C AND BLOOD SUGAR

The following comparison between HbA1C and blood sugar levels gives you an idea of the relationship between test results and blood sugar levels. In the test on page 218, the normal range is 4 to 6 percent. Ask for the normal range and equivalents for the tests that you take, because these vary according to how laboratories interpret their results.

Table 10.3   Comparing Hemoglobin A1C and Blood Sugar

HbA1C	Blood Sugar(mg/dl)	Blood Sugar(mmol/L)
4%	60	3.33
5%	90	5.00
6%	120	6.66
7%	150	8.33
8%	180	10.00
9%	210	11.66
10%	240	13.33
11%	270	15.00
12%	300	16.66
13%	330	18.33

LIPID PROFILE

A lipid profile measures the levels of such fats as cholesterol, triglycerides, and other lipoproteins in the bloodstream. The American Diabetes Association recommends that you receive this test every year. Your lipid profile needs to be periodically evaluated by your doctor because these test results have a direct relationship with possible heart and vascular complications, such as hardening of the arteries.

A lipid profile will show abnormally high levels of fats, or lipids. The results may be used to plan strategies for control. If you have problems controlling fat levels, greater attention to blood sugar testing and control, plus redoubled efforts in the areas of diet and exercise, are often recommended. Lipid-lowering drugs may also be prescribed.

Table 10.4   Lipid Levels

Cholesterol Levels:

<200 mg/dl (11.11 mmol/L)	Desirable
200–239 mg/dl (11.11–13.28 mmol/L)	Borderline
>240 mg/dl (13.33 mmol/L)	High

Low-Density Lipoprotein Levels:

<130 mg/dl (7.22 mmol/L)	Desirable
130–159 mg/dl (7.22–8.83 mmol/L)	Borderline
>160 mg/dl (8.88 mmol/L)	High Risk

High-Density Lipoprotein Levels:

>35 mg/dl (1.94 mmol/L)	Desirable

Cholesterol has gotten an avalanche of media attention in recent years, but remember that cholesterol is not the only reliable indicator of cardiovascular health. As a rule of thumb, cholesterol below 200 mg/dl, or 11.11 mmol/L, is considered good. Desirable levels of low-density lipoproteins, or "bad" cholesterol, are less than 130 mg/dl, or 7.22 mmol/L. Desirable levels of high-density lipoproteins, or "good" cholesterol, are greater than 35 mg/dl, or 1.94 mmol/L. LDL is called "bad" cholesterol because it builds up in the body, whereas HDL actually helps clear cholesterol out of the body. A good ratio of HDL to LDL cholesterols is important. Cholesterol results vary from laboratory to laboratory, so be sure that the same laboratory performs all of your tests. Labs associated with academic medical centers and certified by the Lipid Research Clinics are the most reliable.

Hyperlipidemia, or diabetic lipemia, is associated with poor blood sugar control in Type 2 diabetes. This is reflected in high triglyceride levels.

URINE TESTS

Urine tests that check the level of protein in the urine help your doctor to evaluate your kidney function. You should not have more than a trace of protein in your urine because the kidneys normally recycle proteins. Excessive levels of protein in the urine signal a loss of kidney function. A urine sample should be taken at every visit for the first five years of diabetes, and the results analyzed.

Serum creatinine and blood urea nitrogen concentrations should be measured at least once a year. These are muscle breakdown products that are filtered through the kidneys. Levels of creatinine above 2.0 mg/dl or blood urea nitrogen above 30 mg/dl indicate a need for more frequent monitoring. Elevated levels of these substances indicate a decrease in kidney function. Urine tests should also periodically check for microalbuminuria, which indicates a small amount of kidney damage. A microalbumin test can find levels as small as 20 to 400 mg of protein in the urine, a level of damage which doctors note is still manageable—that is, the damage can be prevented or reversed by medication.

An evaluation of kidney function includes a check of your blood pressure. High blood pressure hastens the progress of kidney problems and other complications of diabetes. If you have kidney problems and high blood pressure, they should be aggressively treated by your doctor.

In addition to urine tests, blood chemistry tests can measure levels of sodium, potassium, calcium, phosphate, and bicarbonate—chemicals that help a doctor assess the functioning of your kidneys, adrenal glands, and pituitary. Normal levels of each are:

Sodium: 135–145 milliequivalents per liter of blood (mEq/L)

Potassium: 3.5–5.0 mEq/L

Calcium: 8.5–10.5 mg/dl

Phosphate: 2.6–4.6 mg/dl

Bicarbonate: 18–23 mEq/L

ORAL GLUCOSE TOLERANCE TEST (OGTT)

The oral glucose tolerance test is not suitable for some people. It involves drinking a solution containing glucose, then periodically taking urine and blood samples afterward. Fasting is required prior to taking this test, which is typically given in the early morning.

Since the oral glucose tolerance test is sensitive and the results difficult to interpret, it is only recommended for pregnant women with positive screening tests and normal fasting plasma glucose levels. This test is *not* recommended for people who have been malnourished for a period of time, have eaten less than 150 grams of carbohydrates per day for more than three days, have been confined to bed for more than three days, or have been experiencing acute medical or surgical stress.

In people without diabetes who take a preliminary glucose challenge test, which involves the ingestion of 50 grams of glucose, blood sugar levels typically climb to about 140 mg/dl, or 7.8 mmol/L, in the first hour, then return to normal. If the results of this preliminary test are positive, a glucose tolerance test should be given as soon as possible. The oral glucose tolerance test involves an eight-hour overnight fast, with periodic blood glucose samples taken in the morning. Frequently, people with diabetes who undergo this test experience symptoms of mild hypoglycemia, including weakness, sweating, or dizziness during the second or third hour.

Glucose Tolerance Test

After an eight-hour overnight fast and after drinking 100 grams of glucose, called a "glucose load," pregnant women may be diagnosed with gestational diabetes if two plasma glucose readings equal or exceed the following:

Blood Sugar	*Test Results As Shown*
Fasting	104 mg/dl (5.8 mmol/L)
1 hour	194 mg/dl (10.8 mmol/L)
2 hours	165 mg/dl (9.2 mmol/L)
3 hours	145 mg/dl (8.1 mmol/L)

FRUCTOSAMINE ASSAY

A relatively inexpensive test, the fructosamine assay checks the level of fructosamines, or sugars bound to certain proteins, that have occurred over the previous seven days to three weeks. This test, like the glycosylated hemoglobin test, measures average sugar levels over a period of time, but the fructosamine assay is most frequently used to check blood sugar levels in pregnant women. Versions of this test have been approved for home use. One company is marketing a meter, similar to a glucose testing meter, that can be used approximately once a week to track changes in blood sugar control over the past two or three weeks.

Table 10.5   **Fructosamine Levels**

Normal	1.4–2.7 mmol/L
Controlled Diabetes	2.0–3.9 mmol/L
Sporadic Control	2.3–5.3 mmol/L
Uncontrolled	2.8–5.0 mmol/L

OTHER SPECIALISTS, OTHER TESTS

The monofilament test for sensation in the feet should be given at every doctor's visit. A foot specialist may also test you to determine if you have poor blood circulation in your extremities. To find these problems (which will show up as variations in your blood pressure) your podiatrist or orthopedist may use *blood pressure cuffs,* like those used to test blood pressure in your arm, but place them on your thigh, calf, ankle, and forefoot. These test results tell your podiatrist how effectively your blood is circulating to important parts of your body, such as your feet and legs. In the special cases in which an artery may need to be reconstructed, a vascular surgeon may give you an *arteriogram.* This test involves injecting a special dye into an artery and taking X rays, which can show where the arteries have become clogged.

Ophthalmologists, or eye doctors, perform most of their tests through visual examinations. A face-to-face examination by an ophthalmologist is considered better than a picture of the eye taken by a machine, which is being substituted for an exam by some health maintenance organizations (HMOs). However, testing for glaucoma, an easily controlled eye problem that affects many people over age forty, involves a test that measures eyeball pressure.

Medical tests are useful to you and your doctor because they chart the progress of your health. Ask about your test results. If you wish, keep a medical file containing your own set of test results. Test results slightly above generally accepted guidelines may or may not be a cause for concern. Unacceptable results should cause your doctor to recommend certain actions, including referrals to medical specialists. The next chapter examines the day-to-day prevention of minor problems, another aspect of self-management.

FREQUENCY OF MEDICAL TESTS

Here are some recommendations for the most important medical tests given by the doctor who is treating your diabetes:

Each visit:

- Blood glucose (finger stick)
- Checking the results of your blood glucose meter against lab test results
- Urine analysis (for protein)
- Blood pressure

At least every six months:

- Glycosylated hemoglobin or Hemoglobin A1C test

At least once a year:

- Lipid profile, including cholesterols and triglycerides
- Blood counts and blood chemistry tests
- Blood and urine tests for electrolytes, blood urea nitrogen, and creatinine; urine testing for microalbuminuria, if complications involving the kidneys are suspected

Chapter 11

VIGILANCE

Good Daily Hygiene Prevents Many Health Problems

~

SELF-MANAGEMENT SUCCEEDS ONE DAY AT A TIME, BUT THINKING AHEAD WILL HELP you prevent many of the problems associated with diabetes. Included in this chapter are recommendations on day-to-day hygiene and prevention. These include strategies to help you maintain a healthy heart as well as healthy feet, eyes, skin, kidneys, and teeth—areas of the body at particular risk. Also included are precautions to take on sick days, when blood sugar almost always goes out of whack.

Good self-management essentially means taking good care of yourself. This involves educating yourself, coordinating your self-management efforts with those of your medical team, adopting a healthier style of eating, and taking action to give yourself a less stressful, more physically active life. Coordinating these diverse elements in a positive way helps you control your blood sugar, and this affects the way you feel.

In addition, taking good care of yourself involves spending a little time each day checking out your body, and taking sensible precautions with your health. A bit of vigilance every day may well prevent or minimize physical problems.

THINGS TO DO EVERY DAY

Every day, examine your body for a few minutes. Look at your feet, skin, teeth, and eyes. These areas can be sites for complications. If you see even minor problems developing in these areas, call the doctor who treats your diabetes and report them. Since diabetes doesn't immunize you against other health problems, don't assume that every ache and pain you have is related to diabetes.

Think of the few minutes it takes to make a daily self-examination as your own personal early warning system. This is particularly true for the feet and skin, which you should check *every day* for any unusual growth, swelling or redness, or cuts or bruises. Note any problems with your eyesight, or with the general look and appearance of your eyes, or anything different in other parts of your body.

As you go about your life, take precautions that can prevent problems. For instance, always wear gloves or protective clothing when doing tasks such as working in the garden. Treat cuts, blisters, and other small medical problems promptly.

If you don't understand how to handle or treat a problem, call the nurse at your doctor's office and ask. Write down what the nurse tells you, and follow these instructions. Be sure to ask what to look for over the next several days, or as healing progresses. Ask how soon you should call back to make an appointment if the problem doesn't go away. Unless you've been instructed otherwise, for minor problems, you should ask to speak with the nurse rather than the doctor. If the nurse can't handle the problem, or if it requires your doctor's attention, the nurse will ask the doctor to call you.

REGULAR DOCTOR VISITS

Regular visits to a foot doctor, an eye doctor, and a dentist are good preventive measures, and a part of good diabetes care. If you aren't automatically referred to a foot doctor or an eye doctor right away, you may have to assert yourself. Gently remind your doctor that you must be referred to medical specialists at certain times. When you bring this up, you may bring the latest recommendations of the American Diabetes Association into the doctor's office with you; they may be obtained by calling that organization's toll-free phone number listed in the "Other Resources" appendix of this book.

"My experience with managed care is that unless you educate yourself about what tests need to be done and when, you may not get those tests done," said an assertive woman who *always* sees the specialists she needs to see. "My doctor may be ready to refer me at one year, but if he doesn't, I'm there to remind him to do it."

Controlling your blood sugar is the best preventive measure of all because of the serious complications of diabetes that are linked to high blood sugar. Maintaining blood sugars within your normal range will accelerate the rate at which you heal; out-of-control blood sugars will slow down natural healing.

In much of the world, weather conditions change drastically throughout the year. Changes in weather mean changes of clothing and lifestyle for all people. As the seasons roll around, plan ahead. Make sure that you have the items you may need, such as moisturizing cream in the winter, and a supply of sunscreen and sunglasses with UV protection in the summer and during ski season. Check the condition of your shoes from time to time, even if you live in the tropics, because shoes with good support and proper cushioning help keep your feet in good shape.

Foot care, heart health, eye care, kidney function, skin care, and dental health are all areas in which you can take preventive action *in addition* to controlling your blood sugar. What follows are some generally accepted recommendations and precautions that you might consider when formulating your personal program of preventive medicine.

HEALTHY FEET

Among the most common medical problems experienced by people with diabetes are problems related to their feet. The human foot was made to walk on grass and dirt, notes Southern California podiatrist Arthur Fass, D.P.M., not on hard surfaces such as concrete, which over time may break down the joints of the foot. Prevention through good daily foot care is important. When you walk around in your daily work or when you exercise, do so in comfortable shoes. If you've received special instructions from your doctor or a foot specialist for treating your feet, follow his or her orders, and promptly report any symptoms that you've been asked to report. Good blood sugar control will help you ward off many foot problems.

The human foot is complex. Each foot is composed of twenty muscles and twenty-six bones. When you walk, each foot becomes slightly longer and slightly wider when it touches the ground. Because your feet are vulnerable, select stable and well-cushioned shoes that match the shape of your feet as much as possible.

It's false economy to purchase cheap, uncomfortable shoes, or to wear shoes that are worn out. If you don't have a good pair of walking shoes or running shoes, begin shopping. Most athletic shoe manufacturers, including Rockport, sell good walking shoes. These shoes may be worn every day. For certain types of exercise, hiking boots and athletic shoes come in various weights and styles. Buy good shoes. Make sure they fit comfortably the first time you slip them on. If you use orthotic devices, make sure that they fit into the shoes you're trying on. *Orthotics,* or shoe inserts, can be helpful in taking pressure off a problem area of the foot, perhaps one that has ulcerated and has been bandaged. If your foot has ulcerated, orthotics can help prevent further ulcerations, provide greater balance, and provide some control that may lessen pain. If you need special shoes, get them.

Rubber soles are often recommended over leather soles because rubber helps to absorb shock. Good shoes insulate the foot from shocks, rocks, and friction. Shoe inserts made by companies such as Spenco can be helpful in absorbing friction from the foot, according to R. Diane Gilman, a doctor of podiatric medicine and an instructor at the University of Southern California. Some podiatrists recommend running shoes over walking shoes because they provide more support for the foot, and they have more toe room. Whatever you select, always wear dry comfortable socks, perhaps two pairs for longer walks. Treat problems when they appear. Foot pain, lower back pain, blisters, bunions, and calluses can be signs of poorly fitting shoes.

Daily inspections are the key to heading off foot problems, which can include infections, ulcers, and deformities. Signs of poor circulation to the feet include:

- dry skin on feet
- loss of hair on feet
- cold feet
- no pulse in your feet
- redness of feet when they are hanging down (or a whitening of skin when feet are raised up above the level of your heart)

Inspect the top and bottom of your feet *every day,* using a mirror or magnifying glass if necessary. A good foot inspection will take less than one minute. If you cannot inspect your feet because your sight is impaired, or you have arthritis or are severely obese, enlist the help of another person, such as your spouse. Ask that person to inspect your feet for you. Watch your feet for obvious signs of trouble, such as:

- redness
- blisters
- cuts
- scratches
- ingrown toenails
- cracks between toes
- discoloration of skin
- any other observable changes

Wash and carefully dry your feet every day, using warm, soapy water. Do not use hot water, which can spread bacteria and cause burns in people with reduced sensations in the feet. Many skin problems in people with diabetes can result from the narrowing of small blood vessels near the skin, called *microangiopathy*. This condition delays healing and increases the chances of an infection from the bacteria and fungi that live on the skin. Tissues can also dry, causing skin to crack and become infected. Good blood sugar control is the key to reducing the susceptibility to infection. Skin creams sold especially for people with diabetes such as Alpha-Keri, Nivea, or Eucerin may be helpful in keeping the skin moist. Most of these creams contain urea; a concentration of 10 to 25 percent urea is probably best, but some trial and error may be necessary. Apply the cream to your heel first and then work it toward the toes, but don't apply between the toes where excess moisture can be a problem. If heels are very dry, try applying the cream before bed for two or three nights and wearing a sock or protective wrap during the night. To prevent athlete's foot, put foot powder between your toes, where sweat and moisture can accumulate.

File your toenails straight across so that they are even with the skin on the toes. Use only an emery board; you can take toenails down a bit at a time. Do not use razor blades, knives, or scissors to trim your toenails because a slip of the blade will break the skin, possibly causing an infection. Avoid over-the-counter medicated corn or wart removers on your feet, because many contain an acid formula that can be harmful to skin (this is why the labels now contain warnings against their use by people with diabetes). Do *not* soak your feet, particularly if you already have sores on them. Don't use a whirlpool. Don't use nail polish, which can promote the growth of fungus under the nails. Rule No. 1 for good foot care is this: If you see something wrong with your feet, such as redness or inflammation, get off your feet for a while.

If you notice a cut or scratch during your daily foot inspection, wash your feet, then apply a mild antiseptic like Bactine. Cover the area with a dry sterile bandage, not Scotch tape or Band-Aids, which can irritate the skin. If the cuts or scratches don't heal within a day or two, call your doctor. Try to stay off your feet until the cuts or scratches heal.

Use common sense when the weather turns very hot or cold, because you may not feel these sensations as well as other people do. *Never* walk barefoot, especially on hot sidewalks. Don't use hot water bottles or heating pads, which can burn the feet. Don't walk barefoot in the snow, or get your feet sunburned. Don't stick your feet into a hot bath without checking it first.

Numbness in the feet, shooting pains, or pins-and-needles type of pain are signs of nerve damage, known as *neuropathy*. If you have neuropathy, inspect your feet more than once a day. Changing shoes and socks several times a day will remind you to make more frequent visual inspections. All shoes basically allow the foot to slide after three to four hours of putting the shoe on anyway, so changing shoes and socks minimizes the chance that blisters and infections will occur.

Don't cross your legs too often, or wear tight elastic hose. And try to stop smoking, especially if you have neuropathy.

If you suffer an ingrown toenail or other foot problem, see a podiatrist or orthopedist; ingrown toenails can become infected and cause severe problems if left unattended. Follow your doctor's orders regarding foot care. Because foot ulcers are difficult to heal, your doctor may ask you to try one of the new pharmaceutical products such as Apligraf, Dermagraft, Fibracol, or Regranex, which are available by prescription and in some cases must be applied by a health-care professional.

The American Diabetes Association recommends that your doctor check for sensation in your feet at least once a year as a part of a comprehensive foot exam. Unfortunately, many doctors forget to do this test unless they are reminded to do it by patients. Simple home test kits have been developed at the Gillis W. Long Hansen's Disease Center in Carville, Louisiana. Home tests are usually accurate, researchers note, but they recommend that any results obtained at home be confirmed by the health-care provider to guard against mistakes.

An estimated 15 percent of people with diabetes will develop a serious foot problem at some time in their lives. Some community-based studies found that foot ulcers occurred in 2 to 3 percent of people with diabetes over the course of one year. Part of the reason for this is that the feet are located at the farthest ends of the cardiovascular and nervous systems. As recommended by your doctor or exercise physiologist, a program of exercise may improve poor blood circulation, but your feet should be checked before and after any exercise sessions. Your doctor may prescribe drugs that help the red blood cells pass through clogged arteries. Not every person with diabetes has *microvascular,* or small blood vessel, disease in the feet, but this is a common site for it to appear.

A HEALTHY HEART

If you are more than 20 percent over your suggested weight, you can automatically lower your chances of having heart disease and high blood pressure by losing weight. Adopting a comprehensive program of self-management, including lifestyle changes, will help prevent heart problems. Exercise, stress reduction, and changes in eating all benefit your heart. These lifestyle changes are *always* preferable to more expensive medical interventions, which carry risks as well as benefits.

Out-of-control blood sugar is a major factor in vascular complications. High blood sugar should be considered toxic when it comes to your ticker. Major risk factors for heart disease in all people are obesity, smoking, and high levels of cholesterol in the blood. Diabetes is another risk factor for heart attacks and strokes, the number one cause of death in Western countries.

The primary indicator of heart and vascular health is your blood pressure, which should be checked every time you visit a doctor. About 50 percent of people with diabetes develop high blood pressure. If your blood pressure is high, your doctor may ask you to lower the amount of sodium, or salt, in your diet, and reduce your weight, both of which will lower blood pressure and reduce the strain on the heart.

In 1997, the American Diabetes Association recommended aspirin therapy for people with diabetes at high risk for cardiovascular disease to prevent a first heart attack or stroke. It recommended aspirin at a rate of 81 to 325 mg per day (a baby aspirin contains 81 mg, an adult aspirin 325 mg). People who have had a heart attack, stroke, or angina or who have a family history of heart disease; smokers; and people who are obese or have high blood pressure are among those considered high risk. People under age thirty and people with active liver disease, a tendency to bleed, and certain other medical conditions are not candidates for aspirin therapy.

Lack of exercise is a major factor in bringing on heart problems, as is cigarette smoking. Nicotine damages the linings of your blood vessels, makes your blood clot faster, and constricts your arteries—factors that can lead to blockages in your blood vessels as well as strokes and heart attacks. Lowering your risk of heart problems is a good reason to stop smoking, something which any person will eventually succeed in doing if they never stop trying to quit. Having a healthy heart involves maintaining an optimum weight and a healthy lifestyle.

HEALTHY EYES

Regular visits to an eye doctor will help you prevent complications involving the eyes. See an ophthalmologist immediately after being diagnosed with diabetes, or when your doctor or optometrist recommends it. After the initial examination, you should see an ophthalmologist once a year, or more frequently if you have eye problems.

Good control of blood sugars slows the development of eye complications, and often prevents the most severe problems. A research study published in *The Journal of the American Medical Association* in 1989 showed that people with diabetes who maintained good control, defined as blood sugar levels within 10 percent of normal, experienced no eye damage during the course of the study. In the same study, when blood sugars ran consistently higher than 50 percent of normal, some 37 percent of the subjects experienced retinopathy or eye complications.

Because the common cold and the flu can be carried to the eyes by the hands, be sure that you wash your hands before you touch the areas around your eyes if you are sick. Always wash your hands before putting in or taking out contact lenses.

Some ophthalmologists believe that eye exercises, such as looking into the distance periodically when doing close work, reduce eyestrain. Sunglasses that protect the eye from ultraviolet rays are recommended when you're in bright sunlight, on the ocean, or in the snow.

If your eyesight is failing, or if your eye swells up, call your doctor right away and ask for an appointment or a referral to an eye doctor. See an eye doctor immediately if you lose your vision, or if you have acute pain in your eye. Another symptom that needs immediate attention is the sensation that a curtain is being lowered in the eyes. In all of these cases, insist that your eye doctor see you right away.

Two studies published in *The Journal of the American Medical Association* found that age-related damage to a central part of the cornea, called the macula, is twice as common in smokers than in nonsmokers.

HEALTHY KIDNEYS

The kidneys are the janitors of the body, filtering out waste material from the blood and sending it through the bladder and urethra to exit the body in the form of urine. The kidneys work by moving blood through a series of tiny little tubes called *nephrons,* at the end of which are small bunched blood vessels called *glomeruli* that actually do the filtering. The glomeruli eliminate harmful substances containing nitrogen, and reclaim and recycle valuable proteins.

Every time you visit the doctor who's treating your diabetes, you should be tested for protein in the urine, and for other signs of kidney damage. Even if you have lost a bit of kidney function, you can greatly slow down the deterioration of your kidneys by maintaining good blood sugar control—eating healthy foods, exercising, and taking your medications. Working with your dietitian to develop a proper diet, which may be low in sodium or low in protein, is a particularly important part of lowering blood pressure, which takes stress off your kidneys.

When pampering your kidneys, don't forget that old staple of dietary advice—drink plenty of water. Drinking a lot of clear, clean, calorie-free water every day will help prevent many kidney and urinary tract problems. Drinking more water may make you a little more physically active, trotting back and forth to the bathroom, and you'll flush harmful bacteria and waste materials out of your system before they can cause serious problems.

HEALTHY SKIN

Skin problems can be caused by high blood sugar damaging the tiny blood vessels that nourish the skin, reducing the availability of infection-fighting white blood cells. Infections of the skin can be more numerous in people with diabetes, and slower to heal.

To maintain healthy skin, avoid soaking the body for long periods of time because this may cause dry, cracked skin. On the other hand, washing and carefully drying the skin every day will help prevent infections.

Severe sunburns are physically stressful to the body, and can substantially raise blood sugar levels. All people should avoid excessive sunlight; if you must go out in the sun, protect your skin with a sunscreen of at least 15 SPF. In the summer, check for skin rashes, particularly in the folds of your skin. Good skin care for all people means avoiding exposure to excessive wind and weather.

Extremely dry skin can be caused by dehydration, a result of not drinking adequate fluids, being ill, or having poor blood sugar control. Achieving better control of blood sugars will minimize this dryness. If your skin remains dry, try a moisturizing skin lotion containing lanolin. *Always* drink adequate water during the day. And drink more water than usual when you exercise.

HEALTHY TEETH AND GUMS

Brush your teeth at least twice a day, and floss once each day, taking care to pull the floss a bit below the gum line. People with diabetes should see a dentist or periodontist at least every six months. Regular visits can help prevent infections in the teeth and gums. Be sure to tell your dentist and the dental hygienist who cleans your teeth that you have diabetes.

More frequent dental visits are recommended for people with diabetes, particularly those who are older. This is because diabetes can slow the rate of healing from infections anywhere in the body, including the mouth. Excessively high levels of glucose in the blood actually nourish the bacteria that live in the mouth, allowing them to multiply more rapidly. And the thickening effect that diabetes has on the blood inhibits the normal infection-fighting abilities of white blood cells.

Problems to watch for include *gingivitis,* or periodontal disease, which occurs around the teeth without pain in the gums. Periodontal disease results when bacteria grow between your teeth and gums over a long period of time. It is sometimes first noticed when you brush your teeth, and see blood on the toothbrush, or when your dentist notices that your gums are discolored (a result of the infection). Bad breath can be another indicator of periodontal disease. Sometimes a dentist first suspects the presence of diabetes and recommends that the patient see a doctor.

Periodontal disease occurs more frequently in people who have diabetes, and in older people in general. It is normally treated with oral surgery, followed by regular deep cleanings. If untreated, periodontal disease results in bone erosion and eventually loss of teeth. Periodontal disease should be taken care of for the simple reason that it can make it more difficult to deal with diabetes. Infections in the mouth rile up your blood sugar, but having periodontal disease treated will help you control it. Brushing your teeth twice a day with flouride toothpaste, flossing once a day, and avoiding sugary foods will help you avoid gum disease, as will good blood sugar control.

A fungal infection called *thrush* is also more common in people with diabetes, particularly those who smoke or wear dentures, but can be treated with medication.

SICK DAYS

You'll have to handle yourself with special care on the days that you are sick. When you have diabetes, your body is greatly affected by illness. Sickness will make your blood sugar rise, sometimes to unusually high levels.

Call your doctor any time you have an illness that lasts more than twenty-four hours, when your temperature exceeds 101 degrees F, or when you are vomiting and can't keep down liquids, foods, or medicine. If possible, be prepared to tell your doctor the time and results of your latest blood sugar tests, your temperature, and how much food and liquid you are taking.

Even a minor illness such as the common cold or the flu triggers the release of certain hormones that cause the liver to release additional glucose into the bloodstream. These hormones impede the action of insulin, raising levels of blood sugar.

As a precaution, do not exercise when you are sick. Follow your meal plan and drink extra fluids, because your body will need plenty of nourishment to fight off disease.

If you take insulin, immediately report any illness to the doctor who treats your diabetes. You may require more insulin than usual when you are sick. If you take a diabetes medication, do not miss taking a dose; ask your doctor if you should increase the amount you take when you are sick.

When you are ill, try to monitor your blood sugar every three to four hours, or ask someone to do your blood testing for you. Ask your doctor what blood sugar test results should prompt you to call. Over 300 mg/dl, or 16.66 mmol/L, is probably a concern.

Drinking more liquids than normal is important to prevent dehydration when you are sick. Since your kidneys won't be able to handle all the excess glucose, it will spill out into your urine. You'll urinate more

SEVEN REASONS TO STOP SMOKING

1. Smoking raises blood sugar.
2. Smoking raises blood pressure.
3. Smoking cuts the amount of oxygen reaching body tissues, leading to heart attack, stroke, stillbirth, and other dangers. For instance, the risk of dying of cardiovascular disease is three times higher among people with diabetes who smoke.
4. Smoking damages blood vessels, and can lead to blood vessel disease or foot infections.
5. Smokers are more likely to get nerve damage or kidney disease.
6. Smoking makes limited joint mobility more likely.
7. Smoking can cause cancers of the mouth, throat, lung, and bladder.

frequently, and this will pull additional fluids out of your body and dehydrate you. *The Joslin Guide to Diabetes Care* suggests that you guard against dehydration by drinking a cup, or 8 ounces of fluid every half hour or so, alternating salty fluids such as broth or bouillon with low-salt liquids such as water. If you can eat, follow your meal plan but substitute sugar-free liquids such as water for other fluids. If you can't eat, the *Joslin Guide* suggests that you alternate foods containing sugar, such as fruit juices, Jell-O, and Popsicles, with sugar-free drinks.

HYPERGLYCEMIC-NONKETOTIC COMA

The most serious concern during illness is *hyperglycemic-nonketotic coma,* a *hyper-nonketotic coma,* or simply a *diabetic coma.* It's brought on by a major physical stress to the body, such as surgery or infection, which causes a dangerous combination of high blood sugars, insulin deficiency, and excessive urination, resulting in serious dehydration. Undiagnosed diabetes, or reactions to certain drugs, may also trigger the onset of this acute complication.

A hyper-nonketotic coma comes on quite slowly, usually over a period of days or weeks. It's most common in older people; the average patient who experiences it is sixty years of age. Blood glucose readings average 1,000 mg/dl. This condition greatly upsets the normal balance of chemicals inside the body, and in the most severe cases can lead to death. Medical treatment involves hospitalization and aggressive replacement of the fluids lost by the body, including potassium, which is typically depleted, and sometimes supplemental insulin.

Call your doctor immediately if you experience the symptoms of this condition when you are sick—excessive urination, great thirst, hunger, drowsiness, nausea or vomiting, abdominal pain, mental disorientation, or shallow rapid breathing. Call your doctor *immediately* if your blood glucose levels test higher than 600 mg/dl, which is one characteristic of this life-threatening complication. If you cannot reach your doctor, proceed to a hospital emergency room and explain your situation.

Taking a little time each day to practice preventive measures and good hygiene will help maximize good health. Vigilance in regularly checking and cleaning the feet, skin, teeth, and other parts of the body can prevent small problems from becoming big ones. Taking care of yourself on sick days is an important part of dealing with the physical aspects of diabetes. And if you become pregnant, the topic of the following chapter, you'll have to take especially good care of yourself.

Chapter 12

PREGNANCY

Taking Good Care of Yourself Prevents Most Problems

~

A NUMBER OF SPECIAL PRECAUTIONS ARE IN ORDER WHEN WOMEN WITH DIABETES become pregnant, or when pregnant women develop diabetes. But the chances of a successful pregnancy are quite good when proper medical treatment is received.

When the twentieth century began, about 27 percent of women with diabetes who attempted to have children died giving birth. Most pregnant women with diabetes lost their babies. Today, due to medical advances, the survival rate for mothers with diabetes is the same as for all women—almost 100 percent. Infant survival rates now exceed 97 percent.

Although babies born to mothers with diabetes are at three times the risk of babies born to mothers without diabetes, good medical care, including a dietary and exercise regimen for the mother, helps produce normal, healthy babies.

GESTATIONAL DIABETES MELLITUS (GDM)

Gestational diabetes mellitus (GDM) is a form of Type 2 diabetes that develops during pregnancy and usually resolves itself after the baby is born. Pregnant women are at greater risk of developing gestational diabetes if they have diabetes in their families, if they weighed more than 9 pounds at birth, if they are obese, if they are over the age of thirty, if they experienced gestational diabetes in previous pregnancies, or if they have had a history of glucose intolerance. Other risk factors for gestational diabetes include frequent miscarriages, recurring urinary tract infections, a history of toxemia, and unexplained stillbirths. Gestational diabetes occurs in 3 to 12 percent of pregnant women, but may be controlled with good medical care and lifestyle changes.

Gestational diabetes occurs because during pregnancy, the hormones produced by the placenta, including estrogen, progesterone, and human placental lactogen, cause insulin resistance, which is characteristic of Type 2 diabetes. Occasionally, routine blood sugar testing during pregnancy uncovers a case of Type 1 or Type 2 diabetes that has not been previously diagnosed.

True gestational diabetes is typically first diagnosed about six months into pregnancy through an oral glucose tolerance test. An early indicator of diabetes is if the pregnant women's fasting blood sugar tests are above 105 mg/dl, or if blood sugar levels two hours after eating a meal exceed 150 mg/dl. If a woman is considered high risk, a glucose tolerance test may be given immediately upon the discovery that she is pregnant, and again at the usual time if the first test is negative.

HEALTHY BABIES

Women who already have diabetes can conceive and deliver healthy babies. Ideally, they should develop and follow a plan to maintain good control of blood sugars before their pregnancies. Vitamin supplements, particularly folic acid, a B vitamin, have been shown to greatly reduce the chances of birth defects. Iron and calcium supplements are also normally prescribed.

Some complications of diabetes, such as retinopathy, can worsen during pregnancy, then return to normal after the baby is born, but should nonetheless be evaluated by medical specialists. Women with Type 2 diabetes who take diabetes pills will be advised to stop taking them and to immediately begin taking insulin, which does not harm the fetus. Insulin requirements often increase dramatically during the pregnancy, but can drop during the final weeks.

BLOOD SUGAR CONTROL

A primary goal of pregnant women with diabetes should be maintenance of their blood sugar levels using diet, moderate exercise, and sometimes insulin. Gestational diabetes should *not* be treated with diabetes pills because they have not been studied or cleared by the FDA for use during pregnancy. It is generally believed that hypoglycemic medications might harm the fetus or result in poor blood sugar control during pregnancy. Good control of blood sugars is necessary for the proper development of the fetus, especially during the first trimester of pregnancy.

Ideally, pregnant women with diabetes are cared for by a treatment team composed of a nurse clinician, a dietitian, a counselor such as a social worker, an exercise specialist, and a team of medical doctors including a diabetologist or an endocrinologist (if the woman knows that she has diabetes before she becomes pregnant). The medical team also includes an obstetrician or a perinatologist (a doctor who specializes in high-risk pregnancies), and a pediatrician or neonatologist (a pediatrician who specializes in the care of newborn babies). Pregnant women with diabetes should visit their doctors more often than women who do not have diabetes.

BLOOD SUGAR DURING PREGNANCY

Ideal blood sugar levels during pregnancy are:

Fasting—60–90 mg/dl
    (3.33 mmol/L)

One hour after meal—120 mg/dl or less
    (6.67 mmol/L)

Two hours after meal—100 mg/dl or less
    (5.55 mmol/L)

A diet plan during pregnancy involves consistent timing of three well-planned meals and three or four snacks, including a bedtime snack. Moderate exercise is usually recommended for all pregnant women, but women with diabetes may have limits imposed on their activities. For instance, pregnant women with diabetes may be asked to limit their exercise to the same intensity and duration at the same time each day, to assure maximum blood sugar control. If blood sugar or ketone levels are too high, insulin will be required.

Pregnant mothers are often asked to check their ketones before breakfast, and before taking insulin if that is part of their treatment. If ketones are present in more than trace amounts for two days in a row, call your doctor. Ketones may indicate that *starvation ketosis* is present. Although it sounds serious, this condition is often remedied by an adjustment in eating schedule, or a change in the composition of the bedtime snack.

Pregnant women should also check their ketone levels when they are sick, even with a minor illness such as a cold or the flu. Some medications prescribed during pregnancy, such as Macrodantin and Pyridium, may cause false positive results in ketone tests. Many doctors advise an immediate check of ketones if the blood sugar is above 200 mg/dl at any time during pregnancy. If blood glucose levels are extremely high, it can result in harm to or the death of the fetus.

Noninvasive tests that pregnant women with diabetes frequently receive include an ultrasound test (including a biophysical profile), a fetal movement counting test done by the mother at home, a fetal heart rate analysis, and an oxytocin challenge test. An amniocentesis is often done in women over age thirty-five. All of these tests monitor the condition of the fetus as it develops. Well-controlled blood sugar at the time of delivery minimizes the risk of complications in the newborn baby.

Breast-feeding is usually recommended, with calcium and iron supplements for the mother. Breast-feeding is delayed if the infant is placed in a newborn intensive care unit; mothers can request breast pumps to stimulate their supply of milk.

Glucose tolerance tests are often given from six to twelve weeks after delivery of the baby to determine if the diabetes has disappeared or stabilized, or if glucose tolerance remains impaired.

If you have had gestational diabetes, even if it disappears after your pregnancy, you have a 90 percent chance of experiencing it again the next time you become pregnant. If you return to an ideal body weight, controlling your weight through exercise and diet, your chances of developing Type 2 diabetes within five to ten years are less than one in four. If you were obese before pregnancy and remain so after pregnancy, you have a 60 percent chance of developing Type 2 diabetes within five to ten years.

Gestational diabetes may usually be controlled through good medical treatment. The emotional and social aspects of diabetes, which affect all people, are dealt with in the next chapter.

Chapter 13

MENTAL HEALTH

A Look at the Social and Psychological Aspects of Diabetes

~

EMOTIONAL AND SOCIAL SUPPORT IS IMPORTANT TO ALL PEOPLE. AFTER A DIAGNOSIS of diabetes, however, you may face some new problems in your family or social circle. You may need to develop better communication skills to handle the new feelings and issues that may arise. Psychological treatment or counseling may help. A diabetes support group may also help you cope; this chapter explains what support groups are and how to find a good one. Even with supportive family members and friends, you may occasionally face diabetes burnout. During these times, you need to identify problems in your self-management routine, address them, and move on with your life.

Without thinking about it, most people develop a network of people with whom they interact and who support them—their own personal support system. Your family, friends, neighbors, coworkers, the people in your religious life or community club—even the people whom you see only occasionally, such as your barber or hairdresser—may support you in ways that are important to you. A diagnosis of diabetes, or your own attitudes about diabetes, may cause emotional ripples to spread out within your personal support system, and temporarily upset the balance of your life. Be prepared for this.

You may experience great emotional distress at certain times, with strong feelings such as loneliness, anger, fear, and depression. Sometimes you may feel overwhelmed, fighting to cope with all the feelings and changes in your life as you adjust to the idea of having—and managing—diabetes. Frustration, despair, rage, even the feeling that you have forever lost control over your life are experienced by many people with a chronic illness. Since diabetes requires more of your own participation than almost any other disease, you may feel that you *must* stay on top of it twenty-four hours a day. The sheer volume of these demands may set you up for feelings of guilt and disappointment. Strong emotions intensify stress; constant stress can cause an emotional riot. Whacked by powerful feelings, you may struggle to control your blood sugar, and return stability to your life.

Connections with people who know you and care about you, in your family or your community, are important in maintaining a healthy life. Research shows that people who interact with others live longer, healthier lives than those who lead lonely, isolated lives. Two lengthy research studies, one conducted near San Francisco, California, and the other in Eastern Finland, studied the effects of social isolation on men and women over a period of five years or more. Both studies found that people who felt socially isolated were 200 to 300 percent more likely to die of various causes compared with those who felt part of a community. Even when the research subjects had a risky medical condition, such as high blood pressure, their membership in a church, synagogue, or social club provided substantial protection from heart disease. Another study of people aged sixty-five and older, conducted at Duke University Medical Center in Durham, North Carolina, found that those without social support were more than three times as likely to die during the course of the research than the subjects who had social support. No one lives forever, of course, but these and many other research studies show that it's healthy to maintain social and emotional links with others, and to participate in community life.

At all times, remember that you are *more* than a person who has a disease. You are *not* your diabetes. Many aspects of self-management of diabetes become routines after a while, requiring only a few minutes here and there. To live a successful life, with or without diabetes, it helps to have a positive self-image, an appreciation of what you have, a good attitude, and the belief that you can help and empower yourself. In the drama of our lives, we all play many roles—parent, child, brother, sister, friend, coworker. It helps to have emotional and social support from the other players on the stage, but such support is not always forthcoming.

FAMILY PROBLEMS

According to Steve Degelsmith, a Los Angeles marriage and family therapist who facilitated support groups for people with diabetes for several years, family relationships can run awry in two ways when a family member develops diabetes:

OVERINVOLVEMENT

Family members may see the person with diabetes as someone who needs to be rescued, someone so fragile that she can't care for herself. This can create a powder keg of strong feelings and resentments on both sides. To the person with diabetes, family members may seem to be turning into parents. They may become the "diabetes police," monitoring your food and lifestyle choices to an extent that is humiliating to you. If you're the person with diabetes, you may feel that you're being lectured everywhere you turn. If your family members become overinvolved in your self-management program, you may lash out at them with a burst of anger, or fall into a depression. Overprotection erodes intimacy and trust, and creates a buildup of antagonism, guilt, anger, resentment, and other strong feelings that are not easily resolved.

UNDERINVOLVEMENT

On the other hand, family members may not be as involved with the person who has diabetes as that person would like. Certain family members may back off because they can't deal with their own unresolved feelings about being abandoned, about supporting other people, or about disease. The faithful caregiving spouse may sometimes get tired of taking you to the doctor's office and hearing you complain. Underinvolvement may also spring directly from the person with diabetes, who projects an air of "I don't need help," causing other family members to back off because they believe that their help isn't wanted or needed.

Financial squabbles about who maintains the insurance or who pays which bills may become bones of contention, and lead to feelings of resentment, isolation, or depression. Some people try to escape from these situations by obsessively throwing themselves into being good parents or grandparents, or taking on a recreational activity. Some even become workaholics, which may avoid some conflicts for awhile, but doesn't resolve any emotional issues. Variations on this scenario can arise in other social situations or at work.

SOCIAL SUPPORT

In almost every family, Degelsmith believes, better communication skills would help. Most people are only partially skilled in this area. When the feelings that accompany a chronic disease such as diabetes are added to the emotional mix, honest communication becomes both more important and more difficult. Every family member needs to develop the ability to tell other people how they feel and what they want, and to speak up when their feelings are hurt, all in an effective but nonjudgmental way. Every person can develop a greater ability to listen. The most productive actions and words are probably those that express love, care, and concern. Effective support is respectful and sympathetic.

You may not always get all of the emotional or social support that you need. Family members who are emotionally upset are often difficult to approach, and their responses can be unpredictable. They may be sitting on a different kind of emotional powder keg than the one you're on. Remember that anger frequently covers fear. Members of your family may be angry, resentful, or jealous of the attention that you receive (or of the attention they don't receive) because you have diabetes. The same feelings can occur outside the family. In the world of urban singles, for instance, friends function much like extended families; a dispute with a friend may hurt you as deeply as a problem in your family.

Hold on to your hat. You may feel as if you've climbed onto an emotional roller coaster. Recognize that you may have emotional ups and downs—give yourself permission to experience your own tempestuous emotions. All of them will pass. Hold on to your sense of humor. Give yourself permission to laugh at the stupid little things in your life that can seem so preposterously important at first. Be as patient and as kind with yourself as you are with other people.

Outside your inner circle, you'll have to decide who to tell that you have diabetes. You aren't required to tell your medical condition to everyone you meet the moment you meet them. You may wish to never tell certain people, particularly those who gossip about you, or who may sabotage your efforts to keep your weight or blood sugar under control. But keeping your diabetes a secret from everyone you know probably isn't a wise strategy either, because this may make you feel dishonest and guilty, as if you're hiding a terrible secret.

Be as honest and as open as possible. Remember that the way in which you present your diabetes to other people helps shape how they view it.

COMMUNICATION SKILLS

Diabetes may involve grieving, particularly when you are first diagnosed or when complications threaten. Give yourself permission to experience all of your strong feelings. Use stres management techniques, such as those listed in chapter 5, to reduce the negative stress in your life. Talk about your feelings with family members or friends who can listen to you and support you. You can sometimes defuse other people's frustrations by listening carefully to them, then responding honestly and tactfully to what they say. You may need to make a special effort to hear well-intended comments as support, rather than as criticism or unsolicited advice. Living with a chronic disease can also be stressful for your family members and friends, since they may become involved and feel some additional responsibility. This may bring some family members into contact with their own worst fears, such as the fear of being abandoned. If you're the person with diabetes, you will sometimes have to support other people rather than the other way around.

The trick is to assert yourself without getting aggressive or lapsing into passivity. An assertive communications style involves speaking up for things you think are important, asking for what you want directly, saying yes and no when you need to respond that way, and more or less "owning" what you say. This does take some courage and tact, especially if important family members are involved, but assertiveness is a skill that can be learned. If the process seems intimidating, you can use forward planning to work out what you want to say to a person beforehand, thinking of the best time and place to say it to them, and then appropriately communicating your message to them.

Make an effort to communicate some of what you're going through. Listen when people who care about you speak. Try to make your verbal exchanges true conversations, containing genuine exchanges of feelings, rather than lectures, evasions, contests, manipulations, or judgments. Begin sentences with "I feel" rather than "you should."

If you're the person with diabetes, don't forget to share even your small successes with family members or friends who will understand and be appreciative. Sharing good news will help them as well as you.

Honest, effective, two-way communication is a subtle art. It can be a first step toward resolving emotional issues, or at least learning to live with them. Recognizing that you're not honestly or effectively communicating how you feel is a first step. Identifying a particular problem or a pattern of miscommunication can be another. Communicating your concerns in a nonjudgmental way can begin the healing process after the problems are identified. Remember that communication continues over the course of a relationship, rather than ending after one or two remarks.

Initiating a conversation about your medical condition will give other people permission to discuss it. Some individuals won't talk about it unless you break the ice. If you do begin this discussion, some family members or friends may feel that they're being put on the spot. You may have to bring up the subject more than once before they *really* feel that it's all right to talk about it. Others may surprise you by communicating or helping out more than you would expect.

If you ask for assistance from people, be specific. Your family or friends may be able to help by bringing you magazine articles or books to read about diabetes, giving you a ride or accompanying you to the doctor's office, or keeping you company in an exercise class. Children and grandchildren need to understand that they have not somehow caused your diabetes, and that you don't expect them to be able to fix it. Classes on communication skills are offered in many communities, and can be quite useful.

PROFESSIONAL COUNSELING

Your personal support system may not be enough to help you get through the first days and weeks of managing your diabetes, or to deal with any complications. After all, you are simultaneously grieving the loss of your previous state of health and being forced to face your mortality. During difficult times, you may find it useful to visit a mental health professional, or to join a diabetes support group.

Consider seeing a psychiatrist, psychologist, or social worker if you have a depression that won't go away, or if you exhibit frequent and repeated self-destructive behavior, such as going on eating binges or forgetting to take your medicine. Consider seeing a mental health professional when you have a constant sense of being overwhelmed, a sense of helplessness that blocks your ability to learn or to take action, or when you simply can't ask for help from anyone else. Another sign that you need to see a mental health professional is when you participate in negative social situations that hamper your self-management of diabetes. A 1999 study of people with diabetes who suffered from depression compared the results of medical care versus medical care and psychotherapy. Some 85 percent of the group receiving psychotherapy reported feeling less depression, versus 27 percent of the untreated group. People receiving psychotherapy also achieved lower HbA1c levels (9.5 percent versus 10.9 percent).

Personal counseling can help you. Mental health professionals may be valuable members of your health-care team because they can help you sort through the issues that you face, and begin dealing with them. Counseling with a minister, priest, rabbi, or other religious leader can also be quite comforting.

Visiting a support group of people with diabetes can be beneficial. Support groups can extend and strengthen your emotional support system. They give people with diabetes, and sometimes their families, a safe place to address the issues relating to diabetes. At their best, support groups provide a comfortable, secure place where unique feelings may be heard and understood.

SUPPORT GROUPS

Support groups should consist of compassionate, supportive men and women. They exist not only for people with diabetes, but also for people dealing with other life and health issues, such as overeating or cancer. The format for support groups is similar to that employed in group therapy, where several people gather at a particular time to discuss issues of interest to them, under the eye of a trained facilitator. All discussions are confidential. In diabetes support groups, the common bond is diabetes.

Typically, support groups are not limited to the discussion of psychological problems. The best groups make sure to discuss personal successes with diabetes. Group members often support each other in a positive, caring way. Support groups provide a place where people can hear how other people deal with problems, pick up practical tips, and receive encouragement in their own lives.

Fighting the daily ups and downs of diabetes can be a lonely and frightening process. Talking about it with people who are also dealing with these issues can be profoundly helpful. There is comfort in people honestly discussing their problems, and offering each other solace. Support groups give many men and women who participate in them an empowering lift.

"The support I've gotten from the people in this group is really important to me," one woman told her support group.

"I got more information here than I ever got from any doctor," said another man.

Asked what she got out of the group, another woman sighed and replied simply, "Emotional support."

Diabetes support groups are open to everyone with diabetes. They're not for everybody, but they are a godsend for many. Each support group meeting is different because it contains different people. Sometimes, discussion begins on a set topic. Most groups have members who attend every meeting, and others who come from time to time.

To locate a support group in your area, call the local American Diabetes Association. Support groups are sponsored as educational programs by hospitals, clinics, health-care organizations, and individual doctors. American Diabetes Association chapters can provide referrals to support groups or to one-on-one programs run by volunteers. Large cities often have several groups, so find one you like. If no support group exists in your area, you may want to start one; the American Diabetes Association can provide guidance.

HOW TO USE A SUPPORT GROUP

Within a support group, you may be able to build your own smaller network of people to call or meet. Participating in a support group may help you deal with some of your powerful feelings—and your tangible problems. Remember, however, that support groups are not composed of medical experts; they are not intended to be forums for medical advice or psychotherapy.

Ideally, support group facilitators are mental health professionals trained by the American Diabetes Association to understand the medical, psychological, and social issues relating to diabetes. Facilitators should know emergency procedures for any medical or psychological problems that arise. A good facilitator will keep meetings on a supportive keel, stopping any individual who constantly complains or criticizes others. Avoiding medical misinformation is crucial; groups not led by a professional facilitator should have a medical resource person who can be called between meetings to clarify any medical questions that arise.

In the best support groups, people who have "been there" can warn you to avoid trying to do too much too fast, can offer words of encouragement when you set or meet a goal, and can make practical suggestions for managing some aspects of life with diabetes. A supportive group can help a member work through a crisis. People in support groups can even laugh about certain aspects of diabetes, a knowledgeable laughter that you may find nowhere else.

Typically, most people in diabetes support groups have Type 2 diabetes. Groups typically meet in the evening or on weekends, when working people are free to attend. Most support groups are free. A group may be topic oriented, or may provide speakers such as medical doctors who can answer questions. Members should be able to suggest topics for future meetings.

You don't need a referral from your doctor to participate in a support group, although some doctors will happily refer you to one. Unfortunately, some doctors may discourage participation. If you think a support group might help you, make up your own mind. Attend three meetings before you decide whether the group is for you.

In places where support groups do not exist, educational meetings do take place from time to time. Such sessions can be good places to meet other people who are dealing with diabetes. You might be lucky enough to meet somebody who can be your telephone buddy when you simply need someone to talk to. Be on the lookout for people with positive attitudes. Avoid negative people, who may hamper your own efforts to learn and persevere.

DIABETES BURNOUT

It's not uncommon to occasionally feel "burned out" from the constant need to practice good self-management. You'll have days when you just don't want to test your blood sugar, don't want to go to aerobics class, or don't want to avoid your family's favorite dessert. On such days, you don't want to have diabetes, and you don't want to think about it either.

Relief from burnout can sometimes be as simple as allowing yourself to take a holiday from your diabetes for a day or two. But at other times, the reasons for your diabetes burnout may be difficult for you to identify. The first step is to identify problem areas in your diabetes management.

William H. Polonsky, Ph.D., has developed a test to help people identify the areas in which they may be experiencing emotional distress with their diabetes. In the magazine *Diabetes Spectrum,* Polonsky defined diabetes burnout as a feeling of being mentally overwhelmed by the disease, which can itself trigger poor self-management and subsequent physical and mental problems.

To identify your problem areas, you may want to discuss your self-management program with a mental health professional or with a member of your health-care team. The twenty problem areas that Polonsky identifies are:

1. not having clear and concrete goals for your diabetes care
2. feeling discouraged with your diabetes regimen
3. feeling scared when you think about having and living with diabetes

4. uncomfortable discussions or confrontations about diabetes with family members, friends, and acquaintances who do not have diabetes

5. feelings of deprivation regarding food and meals

6. feeling depressed when you think about having and living with diabetes

7. not knowing if the moods or feelings that you are experiencing are related to your blood sugar levels

8. feeling overwhelmed by your diabetes regimen

9. worrying about low blood sugar reactions

10. feeling angry when you think about having and living with diabetes

11. being constantly concerned about food and eating

12. worrying about the future and the possibility of serious complications

13. feelings of guilt or anxiety when you get off track with your diabetes management

14. not "accepting" your diabetes

15. feeling unsatisfied with your relationship with your diabetes physician

16. feeling that diabetes is taking up too much of your mental and physical energy every day

17. feeling alone with diabetes

18. feeling that your friends and family are not supportive of your diabetes management efforts

19. coping with complications of diabetes

20. feeling "burned out" by the constant effort to manage diabetes

DISTRESS AND BURNOUT

Emotional distress related to diabetes is apparently quite common, Polonsky wrote. Approximately 60 percent of the respondents in one of Polonsky's studies had a serious diabetes-related concern; no one in the study reported no negative stress. Worrying about future complications and feeling guilty or anxious when getting off track with diabetes management were the most common complaints. Diabetes burnout can spring from the constant psychological demands and pressures of managing diabetes and sometimes in combination with the other demands and pressures of your life.

If you think that you're flunking some aspect of your self-management program, talk about your problem with the appropriate person on your health-care team, such as your medical doctor or diabetes educator. For example, the weight-loss goals that you've set may simply be too ambitious for you at this time. If so, make new goals that you can realistically achieve. Don't set your sights unrealistically high because this sets you up for disappointments. And don't be too hard on yourself, because negative, self-defeating behavior can foster even more of the same.

If you're slipping into burnout, evaluate where you are. Whenever you think it might help, speak with a mental health professional or a religious counselor, or visit a support group. Employing the stress-management techniques touched upon in chapter 5 may also help.

It may benefit you to keep up with medical advances in diabetes by attending lectures and educational programs covering the basics of good care, the latest medical discoveries, and new treatment techniques. This can freshen up your self-management program, since new ideas can be exciting. You may want to participate in a clinical trial; several are usually underway at any one time—the American Diabetes Association can provide information.

Don't slip into the trap of self-pity. Looking at other people, and the seemingly stress-free, happy-go-lucky lives you imagine that they have, may sometimes throw you into a funk. Not everyone has diabetes, of course, but it is an emotional trap to think that everyone has a better life than you. All human beings have problems. Diabetes is merely a fact of your life. Recognize your own strong feelings about diabetes, accept them, and move on.

The famous writer Robert Louis Stevenson lived an extremely productive life while afflicted by tuberculosis, an incurable disease in his time. "Life," the author of *Treasure Island* observed, "is not a matter of holding good cards, but of playing a bad hand well."

The psychological and social aspects of diabetes are important, and they can affect your self-management. Problems can include either over-involvement or underinvolvement of family and friends. Learning to communicate your feelings to the people you care about will help make your emotional ups and downs manageable. In some cases, psychological counseling or a support group may be helpful. If you experience diabetes burnout, identify the areas in which you are having problems, and look for help in the appropriate place. Among the changes you may experience are the effects of diabetes on your finances, the topic of the next chapter.

Chapter 14

MONEY

How to Manage the Financial Aspects of Diabetes

~

THIS CHAPTER COVERS SOME OF THE FINANCIAL ASPECTS OF DIABETES, SINCE EVEN perfectly controlled diabetes costs money. Many treatment costs you can anticipate and manage to some extent. If you have health insurance, it will typically pay a major portion of many of the costs that you may incur, although all costs are never covered. A list of things to check for in your policy after you have been diagnosed with diabetes is included in this chapter, as are suggestions for dealing with insurance companies, health maintenance organizations, and Medicare. Getting new insurance, switching carriers, and suggestions on other ways to pay the costs of diabetes are also included.

Diabetes is time intensive for both the people who have the disease and for the doctors and other health-care providers who treat and educate patients. Dealing with diabetes for your entire life drives up treatment costs.

ESTIMATED COSTS OF DIABETES

Ongoing Costs

MEDICAL TREATMENT	ESTIMATED COST PER YEAR*
Diabetes specialist, four visits @ $50–$85 each	$240–$340
Eye doctor visit and exam, one @ $100–$150	$100–$150
Foot specialist visit and exam, two @ $85–$150	$170–$300
Glycosylated hemoglobin test, two @ $40–$50	$80–$100
Lipid/cholesterol panel, one @ $40–$50	$40–$50
Test strips	
two per day @ 50¢–$1 apiece	$365–$730
four per day	$730–$1,460
Diabetes pills	
No insurance (generic and brand name)	$182–$1,015
Insurance co-payments of $5–$10/month	$60–$120
Insulin, one bottle/month @ $15–$20	$180–$240
Syringes @ $17–$25/pack of 100	$50–$100

Occasional Costs

OTHER EXPENSES	ONE-TIME COST
Blood glucose meter	0–$150
Food scale	$10–$50
Glucose tablets	$1.50 per 6
Insulin cooler	$10–$25
Insulin disposal containers	$4 per 100

* Actual costs will vary from these estimates.

The National Diabetes Information Clearinghouse estimates that the costs of treating diabetes, including lost productivity from missed days at work, totals about $92 billion per year in the United States. According to a consensus statement issued by the National Institutes of Health, the costs for dialysis as a result of kidney failure in people with diabetes totals more than $1 billion per year; these costs are expected to increase over the next several years.

Even perfectly controlled diabetes can cost $1,000 to $2,000 per year, not including reimbursements from health insurance. As shown in the table on page 264, greater costs are incurred when you factor in the frequency of doctor visits, the cost of medications for diabetes, and the costs of supplies. Four visits to the doctor who treats your diabetes, one visit to the eye doctor, and two visits to a foot specialist each year are recommended by the American Diabetes Association, as are two glycosylated hemoglobin tests and at least one lipid profile. The services of a dietitian, an exercise physiologist, a mental health professional, and other medical specialists may be partially covered by insurance.

Some of the costs of diabetes treatment are covered by most health insurance policies. Most routine medical costs, such as doctor visits, medicines, and laboratory tests, should be covered by insurance. A portion of the costs of a home glucose testing meter and supplies may be covered. Complications greatly inflate total medical expenses, but coverage by health insurance or government programs may soften this financial blow.

As with any purchase, shopping around will save you money on items that you must purchase out of your own pocket, since costs of items vary from pharmacy to pharmacy. Rebates are offered on many glucose testing meters, and a few are practically given away. If you are a regular customer who buys many medications, you can sometimes negotiate discounts with pharmacies on medications and supplies. Some insurance companies have special discount arrangements with certain pharmacies. Some mail-order houses specialize in diabetes supplies.

Several of the first-generation diabetes pills are available in generic form, which can be 70 to 90 percent less expensive than brand name medications. Insulin syringes and lancets may be bought in bulk and be reused to cut costs, although sensible sanitary precautions must be taken to keep the needle points protected and clean.

LIFESTYLE COSTS

When you are referred by your doctor, the services of a diabetes educator may be covered by insurance. The services of a registered dietitian are covered by many insurance plans on a case-by-case basis. The services of an exercise physiologist are usually not covered, although a few plans still pay for them. The services of a mental health professional may be covered within certain limits.

The doctor who treats your diabetes may work with a particular diabetes nurse-educator, or refer you to an educational program. Although diabetes education is necessary and cost efficient, the costs of such programs conducted outside your doctor's office may not be covered by health insurance, Medicare, or Medicaid. Take advantage of any educational programs available to you through your health-care provider. If you have not been through an outpatient program that teaches how to manage the day-to-day aspects of diabetes, consider paying for such a program out of your own pocket since most are inexpensive—and a good investment in your health. You can locate a local diabetes educator or an educational program by calling the toll-free number for the American Association of Diabetes Educators, listed in the "Other Resources" appendix. Watch for lectures and panel discussions on diabetes treatment offered through clinics, hospitals, universities, health-care organizations, or your local chapter of the American Diabetes Association.

Except for the services of a nutritional consultant or a registered dietitian, out-of-pocket meal costs could actually decline if a healthier eating style is adopted by the whole family. Avoid the more expensive processed foods by incorporating home cooking and unprocessed whole grains, fresh fruits, and vegetables to replace those TV dinners. A food scale, some measuring cups, and a few good cookbooks are all modest, one-time expenses.

Out-of-pocket expenses for adopting a more physically active lifestyle can be as modest as fifty or sixty dollars for a good pair of walking shoes, or a few dollars for an exercise class. The cost can rise to thousands of dollars per year if you wish to invest in a sports club membership, regular sessions with a personal trainer, special vacations such as cross-country skiing trips, or home exercise equipment.

If you need to see a psychologist, psychiatrist, or social worker, insurance may pay a portion of these costs, particularly if the therapy is short term. Many communities have mental health clinics where clinicians will see you at low cost; fees are based on a sliding scale according to the client's income level. In cities, low-cost psychological counseling can be found at clinics run by colleges and universities. Some private therapists will accept less than their normal hourly rates if you explain that you do not have insurance coverage. Ministers, rabbis, and other religious leaders counsel their members. Support groups affiliated with the American Diabetes Association do not charge a fee, although remember that support groups are not a substitute for therapy.

Miscellaneous costs never covered by health insurance may include new—and smaller—clothes if you lose weight, travel to and from the doctor's office, parking fees, and subscriptions to magazines or newsletters specializing in diabetes.

COSTS COVERED BY INSURANCE

If you have just been diagnosed with diabetes, you may want to find out which costs your insurance plan will cover. This will help you to plan a budget, since costs not covered by insurance are your responsibility. Each insurance plan is different.

When checking your policy or shopping for a new one, consider your needs to see particular doctors, your out-of-pocket payments for medications and supplies, and coverage for hospitalization and ancillary services. Many patient provider organizations, or PPOs, cover blood testing supplies, including a meter and strips. Health maintenance organizations, or HMOs, cover some supplies. Many health insurance providers offer a pharmacy plan that involves co-payments of $5 to $10 for a thirty-day supply of any prescribed drug. Always ask about deductibles and co-payments, which are your responsibility. Here are some areas to examine, and questions to ask, when looking over or comparing health insurance plans.

DOCTORS' VISITS

Can you keep your present doctor and continue to visit the specialists you've already seen? Can you see a doctor or specialist when you need to see one, or are limits imposed?

DIABETES SUPPLIES

Are needed supplies such as a glucose testing meter, strips, and syringes completely covered? If not, what are the limits of the insurance plan? Does your coverage limit your reimbursement to a specified number of strips per month or per year? Are syringes, meters, and strips covered as *durable medical equipment*—equipment that can be used over and over again? Are all types and brands of meters and strips covered, or only a few? Do you need a doctor's referral for your supplies to be covered? Will these items be covered under the *pharmacy benefits* section of the plan in which a prescription will be needed and limits may apply? Are specific medical requirements necessary in order for your doctor to approve the purchase of any of these items?

DIABETES MEDICATIONS

Can you get all of the medications and prescriptions that you need this year? What are your out-of-pocket costs? Is there a limit, or a *capitation,* on your prescriptions? Are only brand name or only generic medications covered? Is your choice of a pharmacy limited, and if so, how convenient is the available pharmacy? What co-payment is required?

HOSPITAL COVERAGE

If you require hospitalization, are you required to go to a particular hospital? Which doctor will take care of you in that hospital? If you're not sure what type of care you will receive, call the hospital's public affairs office and request a copy of the mission statement, which will help you to understand the emphasis at that hospital. Or walk into the lobby and look around.

ANCILLARY SERVICES

Are services such as physical therapy, dialysis, social services, psychiatry, and chemotherapy covered by the insurance plan? Are there dollar limits or provider limits to these services? Is your use of these services restricted to a certain number of visits per year?

MANAGED CARE

The insurance industry is moving toward managed care due to rising health-care costs. Health insurance was once almost exclusively a fee-for-service model, in which the patient paid a portion of the bill and the insurance company paid the rest, often an 80 to 20 split with the insurance company paying 80 percent. A deductible of perhaps $1,000 per year, the amount you paid out of your own pocket, was imposed, with services beyond that covered according to the policy. Under these plans, you could usually see any doctor you wanted to, or any specialist to whom you were referred.

In the newer health maintenance organizations, or HMOs, the patient pays only a small co-payment of perhaps $5 to $10 for each doctor's visit, test, or procedure. HMOs are organized differently than other insurance companies. The primary care physician acts as gatekeeper for all medical services, referring the patient to specialists such as endocrinologists, ophthalmologists, or podiatrists. This arrangement can sometimes relegate the diabetologist or endocrinologist to the role of consultant, with your primary care physician handling many of your regular visits and tests. This works fine if your primary care physician is experienced in treating diabetes, and understands what good treatment involves. However, the HMO structure becomes a problem when you think you need to see a specialist, but your primary care physician won't refer you. In such a case, you may have to assert yourself to get the referrals. So far, only a few HMOs have "point of service" options that allow you to see a specialist on your own, even if your primary care physician doesn't think it's necessary to refer you.

There are several types of HMOs. The smaller ones involve groups of physicians. Some, like Kaiser Permanente, are large nonprofit organizations. A few such as Blue Cross, which were nonprofit, are spinning off special HMOs and for-profit divisions. Health-care companies and hospitals are merging. Even government programs such as Medicare

are shifting toward the HMO arrangement. The important thing to understand is that not every expense will be covered under any insurance policy. Check what your policy covers, and be prepared to explain your coverage to your doctor if necessary.

You could be lucky enough to get one of the really good doctors in a particular HMO. This doctor should understand diabetes care, and make all of the referrals suggested by the American Diabetes Association's Patient's Bill of Rights at the appropriate time. If this is not the case, ask to see another doctor. If you don't wish to exercise that privilege, perhaps you could help educate your doctor about diabetes. The American Diabetes Association's standards of care criteria are a good place to begin—they're easily available by calling the toll-free number listed in the "Other Resources" appendix at the back of this book. Respect your doctor's training and expertise, but respect yourself too.

Know the standards for good diabetes care and insist on them from your physician. If your doctor says that you need a test or a referral to a specialist and your health plan won't cover it, you can prevail if you are tenacious and assertive. Put your case in writing, and send copies to the appropriate people. Get an appeal started right away, and ask for another hearing if you're turned down. If the issue is important, be prepared to carry your case as high as it will go. If you can't seem to get what you need from the health insurance company's bureaucracy, ask your doctor to support you. If the dispute drags on for too long, and your medical doctor says you need the treatment promptly, consider getting the treatment and paying for it yourself under protest, or putting it in financial limbo by withholding payment until the issue is resolved.

INSURANCE COVERAGE

The first thing you should do when reviewing your health insurance policy is to make sure that your premiums are paid up to date. Ask for the most recent plan booklet from your carrier, and make sure that you understand what benefits are available, so that you can receive all the coverage to which you are entitled. This is not the insurance company's responsibility. If you don't submit a claim in a timely manner for something covered by your policy, some insurance companies won't pay the claim, even if you submit the late claim in writing.

If you know ahead of time what procedures you'll need, you may file for *preauthorization* before receiving medical services. Your request should include the proper preauthorization code numbers, as well as the treatment you expect to have. The insurance company can then tell you in writing how much it will cover for a particular treatment.

If you have a question about what your policy covers, call the insurance company's toll-free claims department hotline, and ask for a supervisor. Many experts say that it's best to politely *ask* for help, rather than to shout and rave at insurance company employees. At times, however, you may need to bravely assert yourself. Whenever you speak with a person at your insurance company over the telephone, write down that person's name, the date you spoke with him or her, and what you were told. Always ask the person you speak with about your coverage to put what he or she tells you in writing. If a written document is not forthcoming, write a letter back to that person spelling out exactly what you understood the person to say, and asking for written clarification if you've misunderstood or misinterpreted anything the person has told you.

You might wish to collect all this information in a *medical records file*. You can keep medical records anywhere, in a small portable filing cabinet or even in an old shoebox. It can be useful to have a central location for all the paperwork related to your medical treatment. You may find this file helpful when working out a dispute with your insurance company, or when you need to locate copies of documents or letters that may help you prove a point. Organized materials can help you evaluate your overall financial costs, and may be useful at tax time, since some out-of-pocket costs not covered by health insurance, such as travel to and from the doctor's office, may be tax deductible.

Request and keep a supply of blank insurance forms on file, if your plan requires you to file such forms for reimbursement. Make copies of all the forms that you submit, as well as all correspondence with the insurance company. Check your medical bills for accuracy, and report any errors.

Insurance reimbursements and payments can be aggravatingly slow. Don't give up if your insurance company won't pay a claim that you believe is legitimate. The office staff at your doctor's office can sometimes be helpful. They can check to see if your claim contained the correct procedure code and diagnosis when it was submitted to the insurance company.

If your insurance problem is difficult to resolve, get on the telephone and speak with your broker or an insurance company representative. If the first person you speak to doesn't want to help you, or doesn't seem to understand what you are saying, ask to speak to that person's immediate supervisor. Continue this procedure until you get a person who will address your complaints. Insurance companies all have procedures to review claims; the company will review your claim if you ask it to follow its procedures. If you strike out, call the state department of insurance, since insurance companies are certified by the states. Write to your member of Congress. Speak with a lawyer. As a last resort, hold a press conference. In most cases, legitimate insurance claims are eventually paid, although it can take a lot of patience and time.

To resolve a dispute with your doctor, call a care manager or benefits supervisor at your HMO. When you call, explain your rationale; the HMO can frequently negotiate with your primary care physician. If the dispute intensifies, however, it may be in your best interest to switch doctors.

Medicare's PPO and HMO members also have the right to appeal decisions about what medical services their HMOs will cover. However, appeals may take six months or longer to be resolved. In 1995, according to Medicare statistics, appeals with Medicare HMOs regarding payment for nursing home care, hospital bills, ambulance bills, and care by a non-plan doctor were settled in the member's favor 25 to 39 percent of the time.

NEW INSURANCE

Insurance companies look at certain criteria when writing policies for people with diabetes. These criteria are designed to minimize the financial risk to the companies.

In California and some other states, for a person with diabetes to even have a chance of being insured, insurance companies require that you be within 15 percent of normal body weight; have a history of good blood sugar control, with a glycosylated hemoglobin test of under 8; and have had no complications. According to an insurance broker who writes many policies for people with diabetes, some insurance companies also like to see regular visits to your doctor (every six months or so) before they will write a policy.

It may not be easy to find new health insurance if you have diabetes. Insurance companies consider diabetes to be "high risk." Most insurance companies consider diabetes a preexisting condition, and will insure you only if they can minimize their own financial risk. If an insurance company considers you to be high risk, you may be offered insurance at the normal rate without coverage for diabetes. Or you may be offered coverage for diabetes at an additional charge.

A few insurance brokers specialize in finding insurance policies for people who are high risk—your local American Diabetes Association may be able to recommend a broker who can help you. High-risk policies are always more expensive than standard insurance.

In some states, high-risk health insurance pools will insure anyone, regardless of health. However, many states limit the number of people that they will insure in this manner, and limit the amount of coverage. HMOs sometimes have "open enrollment" periods when they will accept anyone, regardless of previous medical conditions.

Since the states regulate the insurance industry, laws can vary considerably from one state to the next. One Western state has passed a law that insurance companies can't turn down anyone who applies for insurance. Another state in the East passed a law that all medical supplies required by people with diabetes be covered by insurance policies.

If you are laid off from a job that provided you with insurance coverage, and your former employer has more than twenty employees, your former employer's insurance company is obligated to offer you COBRA coverage. This is insurance coverage mandated by the federal government's Consolidated Omnibus Budget Reconciliation Act of 1985. COBRA coverage lasts for eighteen months, but you must pay the insurance premium yourself, so coverage will be more expensive than what you paid for the same policy before.

If you are covered by a COBRA policy, insurance advisors recommend that you *not* wait until the month before it runs out to shop for more insurance. This is because some insurance policies have a ninety-day waiting period before you can be treated for a preexisting condition such as diabetes.

In the past, the difficulty of securing new health insurance almost forced some people with diabetes or their spouses to work for companies longer than they cared to, simply to retain insurance coverage. The Health Coverage Availability and Affordability Act of 1996, known as the Kennedy-Kassebaum Bill, should make it easier for people to retain health insurance coverage when changing jobs or leaving jobs to start new businesses, since insurers are now *required* to renew the policies of people whose coverage might have been dropped in the past. Government jobs often provide health insurance without exclusions for preexisting conditions.

FINANCIAL HELP

According to Maureen Harris, director of the National Diabetes Data Group, government-funded programs including Medicare, Medicaid, and veterans hospitals cover 57 percent of American adults with diabetes, including 96 percent of men and women with diabetes over the age of sixty-five.

The primary health-care program for older people in the United States is Medicare. Medicare is a two-part program that pays some of the expenses associated with diabetes. Medicare Part A provides certain coverage for all qualified recipients. Medicare Part B is optional, and pays for more of your health-related expenses.

There are many special provisions and exceptions in Medicare's coverage of diabetes-related expenses; these are spelled out in the U.S. Health Care Financing Administration's *HCFA Publication 6*. Doctors and hospital billing personnel don't always know exactly which diabetes-related expenses will be covered by Medicare, since many factors affect a Medicare reimbursement, and government regulations are subject to change.

Medicare expenses are billed according to CPT or procedure code numbers. Reimbursements to health-care providers vary based on the insurance carrier, whether services are received as an inpatient or oupatient, what procedure code the expense is billed under, and the amount of other medical expenses billed to Medicare during a particular time period.

If your doctor requires you to take insulin, Medicare will pay for a blood glucose testing meter, as well as for strips and syringes, but won't pay for the insulin. Neither insulin nor diabetes medications are covered under Medicare Part A or Part B. Beginning in 1998, Medicare Part B began providing self-management training, paying 80 percent after you've fulfilled your deductible requirement at educational programs such as those based in hospitals or other locations. As of 1998,

Medicare also pays for test strips, lancets, and blood glucose monitors for people who have Medicare Part B or are in a managed care plan. At the present time, insulin or diabetes pills are only covered under "Medigap"-type policies. Medicare covers 100 percent of approved hospital costs and 80 percent of medical expenses (including dialysis) for most patients with permanent kidney failure. See the "Other Resources" appendix for other sources of help.

Some insurance plans cover only up to the level that Medicare will cover. To receive full coverage of your diabetes-related expenses, a secondary "Medigap" policy such as those sold by the American Association of Retired People, or AARP, must be purchased.

Medicare recipients with diabetes may see a podiatrist, or foot specialist, every sixty days for routine foot care, but if pain is experienced recipients may be seen on an emergency basis. Orthopedic shoes are sometimes covered, depending on how the expenses are billed.

In addition to Medicare, low-income people may have other expenses covered under Medicaid. In many states, Medicaid can help with some expenses for people with diabetes who qualify.

Veterans hospitals treat male and female military veterans at no cost to the patient. Native Americans and merchant marine veterans may be treated free of charge at public health service hospitals.

Teaching hospitals that do research on diabetes often bill for patient services using a sliding scale. Participants in clinical trials that test new diabetes medications or strategies of treatment are sometimes not charged for the medical care that they receive during the trial. Some drug companies have programs that may provide drugs at no cost to people without health insurance, although your doctor must contact the program and enroll you in it. Many of these programs will provide at least a three-month supply of medication to qualified people, which can sometimes be renewed.

If you ask, a few private doctors will treat people with diabetes who have no health insurance for lower fees. If you are eligible for Medicare, ask your doctor if he or she will accept the Medicare assignment, which is the amount Medicare will actually pay for the expenses or treatment in question. Some doctors will accept this amount as their full payment if you ask them.

Sometimes, to save money, supplies such as insulin, lancets, or strips can be bought in bulk, in frequent buyer programs that are less expensive, or from suppliers who offer "buy 10 bottles of insulin, get one free." Pharmacies sometimes offer specials on diabetes supplies, which can be buying opportunities. You can do some price-shopping before making your purchase, utilizing not only pharmacies but also mail-order and Internet suppliers, although medications that are for short term use are best purchased locally. Always make sure you can use the products within the expiration dates, if applicable.

OTHER TYPES OF INSURANCE

Life insurance is usually available for Type 2 diabetics who have fairly normal weight and reasonable glycosylated hemoglobin levels, although the premiums cost more. Protein in the urine, indicating kidney problems, or a recent history of severe complications such as heart problems may completely disqualify you from purchasing life insurance.

Disability insurance is difficult to acquire, and if available, the premiums are often extremely high because of the "high risk" factor. Disability insurance also requires a long waiting period before the policy becomes effective.

Auto insurance premiums can be a little more expensive, since some insurance companies will not write insurance on people with health problems such as diabetes.

INSURANCE: MISTAKES NOT TO MAKE

According to *Diabetes Advisor*, July/August 1999, here are ways to correct five financial mistakes commonly made in dealing with insurance companies:

1. Get prior authorization, especially from cost-conscious HMOs.

2. Keep copies of every letter or claim form you send to the insurance company so you can follow up on unpaid claims, or document what you've done if you must appeal a claim.

3. Read the plan booklet, so you know what your plan covers.

4. Check the statement for errors such as making sure the doctors you actually saw are listed, that you're listed as being in the correct medical plan, and to assure that reasons for denying claims make sense.

5. Don't give up too soon. It's a bureaucracy, and there is an appeal process if a claim is denied. Make sure you make filing deadlines for appeals, and consider asking your state insurance commission for a hearing if applicable. Even if a hearing doesn't allow your claims, you can still try small claims court for relatively small (often under $3,000) claims.

Discrimination against people with diabetes occurs in day care centers, schools, and at work. Very recently, the American Diabetes Association has hired its first national director of legal advocacy to lobby for regulatory, legislative, and litigation changes. According to an article in the July 1999 *Diabetes Interview*, since 1992 more than two thousand people have filed complaints with the U.S. Equal Employment Opportunity Commission alleging mistreatment at work because of their diabetes. The Americans with Disabilities Act offers legal recourse for all people who are discriminated against in companies with fifteen or more workers.

The financial aspects of diabetes can be frustrating if you are required to wrestle with an insurance company to resolve a claim, or to receive all the medical services you need. After you are diagnosed with diabetes, check your policy to see what is covered in the way of doctors' bills, medicines, supplies, and other expenses. Keep records of your correspondence with insurance companies; assert yourself as needed. Some financial help is available to people with diabetes, but even if you have good health insurance you will bear out-of-pocket costs. Medicare and other programs may help. Among the most costly aspects of diabetes to insurance companies are the long-term medical complications that can arise, the subject of the next chapter.

Chapter 15

COMPLICATIONS

Understanding and Treating
the Long-Term Effects of Diabetes

~

THIS CHAPTER LOOKS AT THE COMPLICATIONS OF DIABETES, AND EXPLAINS RELATED medical treatments. Complications that spring from diabetes are almost always traceable to excessive sugar in the blood for many years. High blood sugar over a long period of time slowly weakens certain parts of the body, including the eyes, kidneys, and skin. High blood sugar slowly damages the blood vessels and the nervous system, affecting parts of the body such as the feet, and even sexual function. Since self-management of diabetes doesn't suddenly stop when your health takes a turn for the worst, and since a healthy, physically active lifestyle benefits everyone, exercises appropriate for people with complications are included here. A few things to consider during a hospital stay conclude the chapter.

HEREDITY

Some people can sail through their entire lives without suffering any complications, even if they don't take perfect care of themselves. But a few "good diabetics" suffer complications despite doing almost everything by the book. Most people with diabetes fall between these two extremes. This is because the genes that you have inherited affect your health.

Some people seem genetically predisposed to have certain complications, others predisposed not to. The genes you were born with are not within anybody's control, but you can lower the risk of complications by practicing good self-management and taking good care of yourself. Keep in mind that when you were diagnosed with diabetes, you may already have had the disease for years without realizing it. One prominent Southern California doctor estimates that the average person with Type 2 diabetes has had the disease for an average of eight to ten years before the incidence of diabetes was discovered. You may have sustained some damage from high blood sugar before you were diagnosed.

Good control of blood sugar is the *major* factor in preventing the appearance of complications, and in mitigating some of their worst effects. You can considerably reduce your chances of complications through a program of good self-management. Think of your efforts at good hygiene, and the other preventive measures that you take, as something akin to careful driving. If you drive within the speed limits, there will be less chance of your having an accident than if you always drive too fast.

It's never too late to help yourself by controlling your blood sugars, losing a few pounds, or stopping smoking. Obesity has a correlation with many diseases. Smokers with diabetes are eight times as likely to have complications than will nonsmokers. At any time in your life, you can begin a new and better program of self-management that includes blood sugar testing, stress reduction, lifestyle changes, and medications prescribed by your doctor. Practicing good self-management will help you now and in the future.

LEN'S STORY

A man we shall call Len, forty-one years old, has come through several complications of diabetes with a good attitude.

"I know I'm not going to die from diabetes, and I know that good blood sugar control can stop or minimize the chances of complications," says Len, who works for a major hospital's diabetes education program, which serves people with Type 2 diabetes. "With diabetes, there are a lot of physical battles, and a lot of psychological battles. Sometimes you find you're fighting yourself."

Len was twenty years old and ready to try to pitch his way into major league baseball when he was diagnosed with Type 1 diabetes. The doctor who diagnosed him was quite insensitive, brusquely informing Len that he had diabetes, then hurriedly offering to show him how to inject insulin. Len almost fainted.

"The second doctor I saw was better, " he says. "He told me I had to get my blood sugars under control. I remember him telling me that if I didn't, ten years down the line I'd have problems. I realize now that my blood sugar control after that was not what it could have been."

Len remembers feeling embarrassed after he was diagnosed. None of his friends knew that he had a medical condition or that he was required to eat differently and take insulin to stay alive. He remembers feeling deprived because he couldn't eat the same things that his friends ate.

Len admits that for the first ten years that he had diabetes, he didn't do a good job of keeping his blood sugar under control. It didn't seem to matter. He had a gift for business; he had started one successful business after another. His life was good. He had a nice house and a nice car.

But four years ago, Len's life became a nightmare. First, he was diagnosed with diabetic retinopathy. His eyesight failed; he went completely blind. Then his kidneys failed. He found himself the youngest person in a convalescent hospital, undergoing kidney dialysis three times a week. As his business, house, and cars slipped away, he himself slipped into a depression.

"Many mornings I'd wake up and be disappointed that I didn't die in my sleep," he recalls.

About this time he also broke his leg, a Charcot break, which occurred because his bones had been weakened from the dialysis.

After four long months of believing that he might be blind for the rest of his life, Len had his eyesight partially restored due to the efforts of a good eye doctor, who persisted with treatments and did not write Len off as others had done. Len's broken leg healed. After he received a kidney transplant, his health came back.

Len soon began work as a volunteer at a diabetes education center, where he is employed today. He wears an insulin pump on his belt, and says that he feels better than he has in years because he has better blood sugar control than he has ever had. When he was younger, he says, he would have worried that someone might notice the pump on his belt and reject him. Now, he says, it doesn't bother him one way or the other, since he has come through a difficult time with a new appreciation for life.

"My work is very rewarding," he says. "Sometimes I can relate to our patients on a personal level, because I know what it feels like when your blood sugars are running high. I know what it feels like to go to a birthday party and be the only one there who doesn't get to eat cake. My health is pretty good now, although I have physical limitations. At the end of the work day, I'm pretty tired. But I can't feel sorry for myself, because there are a lot of people worse off than I am."

If you have been diagnosed with any of the complications of diabetes, you may experience additional stress and worry. You may have to grieve all over again, with the attendant emotional ups and downs. As outlined in chapter 5, reducing the level of negative stress in your life can help you control the situation. Eating healthy foods and remaining physically active will help. Remain in contact with the people you care about—and who care about you—including family, friends, and people within your support system. Consider psychological counseling when you feel completely overwhelmed.

Learning more about your medical condition may give you a greater feeling of control. Many improvements in medical treatment have occurred in the past several years, and more advances are on the way. If you experience complications, the doctor who treats your diabetes will probably refer you to a specialist. You may undergo additional tests, and even spend some time in the hospital. All the medicines you take should be prescribed by a doctor who is knowledgeable about your medical condition. Any new specialist you see will ask what medications you are taking. Write down a list of what you take and when you take it, and present the list to any new doctor you see.

POSSIBLE LONG-TERM COMPLICATIONS

Possible complications of diabetes discussed in this chapter include problems with the blood vessels (*vascular* problems) and various problems with the feet, eyes, nerves, and skin, as well as kidney, urinary, and sexual functions. This information is background material, not medical advice. The ultimate authority on your medical care is, of course, your own doctor.

VASCULAR COMPLICATIONS

Diabetes affects the small and large blood vessels. Driven by the rapid beating of your heart, your *cardiovascular* system includes a *vascular* system consisting of many miles of veins, arteries, and small blood vessels, called capillaries. If your heart stops beating, or if major blood vessels clog up, you could die.

Heart attacks are a prime cause of death in middle-aged people with Type 2 diabetes, who have death rates two to four times higher than do middle-aged people without diabetes. A recent study showed that between 35 and 50 percent of heart attack victims had abnormal blood sugar levels at the time of the attack.

The cardiovascular system is compromised by high levels of glucose and fats in the blood, much as plumbing pipes are slowly encrusted by the mineral deposits in tap water. Fortunately, the lifestyle changes you make to control diabetes, such as good diet and regular exercise, are the same lifestyle changes recommended to reduce heart disease.

Large blood vessel, or *macrovascular*, complications can affect the brain, heart, legs, and feet in people with diabetes as well as in older people in general. Small blood vessel, or *microvascular*, disease can lead to problems with the eyes, skin, kidneys, and nerves, and can cause slow healing.

Vascular problems are almost all related to *atherosclerosis*, a hardening or stiffening of the arteries that results from a buildup of deposits along blood vessel walls. This can trigger a heart attack, which doctors call a *myocardial infarction (MI)*. A sharp pain known as *angina* can occur if the arteries supplying oxygen to your heart muscle are blocked. A *stroke* occurs when a blockage of blood vessels occurs in your brain. A blood clot built up in the brain is called *thrombosis*. A blood clot in the body that breaks off and travels to the brain is called an *embolus*. Blood vessels may *hemorrhage*, or bleed into surrounding tissues.

The condition of high fat levels in the blood is known as *hyperlipidemia*. *Atherosclerotic heart disease* results from fat-clogged blood vessels. The combination of high blood pressure, insulin resistance, and high levels of fats such as HDL cholesterol in the blood is sometimes called *Syndrome X,* or *insulin resistance syndrome.* As many as one out of four Americans have Syndrome X, which increases the risks of atherosclerotic heart disease. High levels of homocysteine, an amino acid, are also increasingly believed to factor into incidences of heart disease.

A prime indicator of heart health is your blood pressure, which should be checked every time you visit a doctor. Between 60 and 65 percent of people with diabetes have high blood pressure. Glucose and fats cause the blood vessels to constrict. Smoking is hazardous because nicotine causes all of your blood vessels to constrict, including those leading to the heart, brain, hands, feet, and skin. Your doctor or a heart specialist, called a *cardiologist,* may ask you to lower the amount of sodium, or salt, in your diet, quit smoking, and reduce your weight, since all can lower blood pressure. Very high blood pressure is dangerous, and should be treated.

As needed, medications may be prescribed by your physician. For many people with diabetes, medicines that control blood pressure such as calcium channel blockers, angiotensin converting enzyme, or ACE, inhibitors, and alpha blockers are preferred to the diuretics and beta blockers often prescribed to control blood pressure in people without diabetes. Diuretics and beta blockers actually *decrease* insulin sensitivity in people with diabetes, and can contribute to impotence in men. Note that heart and blood pressure medicines may be discontinued if the problems are brought under control through such methods as weight loss—another reason why it's a good idea to get your blood pressure checked every three months if you have experienced any cardiovascular complications.

Heart-healthy exercise: Most older people have some level of atherosclerosis, whether or not they have diabetes. Aerobic exercise may help control high blood pressure. For a healthy heart and circulatory system, an aerobic exercise such as walking, bicycling, or swimming is recommended because these activities utilize the large muscle groups. Isometric exercises, in which the muscles push against themselves and don't move, are *not* recommended if you have heart or high blood pressure problems. Also *not* recommended for people with high blood pressure are weight-lifting exercises that use only the arms. Recommendations made by Dr. Claudia Graham and her coauthors in

The Diabetes Sports and Exercise Book are the basis of many of the exercise recommendations in this chapter. However, you should *always* check with your doctor before beginning any new program of exercise, particularly when any complications from diabetes occur.

FOOT COMPLICATIONS

People with diabetes spend more days in the hospital with foot infections than with any other complication. Untreated foot infections are dangerous because they can turn into gangrene, a putrefaction of soft tissue that can necessitate the amputation of a toe, foot, or leg. People with diabetes are much more likely to have a complication involving gangrene than will the general population. An estimated 54,000 lower-extremity amputations are performed each year in the United States because of diabetes. The probability of a person with diabetes experiencing an amputation during his lifetime is less than 1 percent. However, authorities estimate that the number of amputations could be decreased by half through proper professional care. In addition to peripheral neuropathy, other risk factors for amputations include insufficient blood flow to the extremities, foot deformities, stiff joints, calluses on the feet, and a history of ulcers on the feet or a previous amputation. Good blood sugar control lessens the chances of any complication. And new surgical techniques, such as grafting new or synthetic blood vessels onto clogged blood vessels that carry blood to the feet, can prevent amputations that once were unavoidable.

Foot problems occur primarily because of poor blood circulation to the feet. Poor circulation is a result of arteries in the legs and feet becoming clogged with plaque (atherosclerosis). Arteries also become somewhat less flexible, partially as a result of high blood pressure and excess weight, which increases triglyceride levels. *Claudication* is another effect of reduced blood circulation, which develops in the calf or another part of the leg when muscles don't get enough blood, creating pain or cramps when walking or a deep ache when the foot is at rest. Many people with diabetes have a diminished ability to feel sensations in the foot, a nerve-deadening complication called *neuropathy,* which can decrease the sensation of pain. This is why it is important to examine your feet on a daily basis, even if they don't hurt, as chapter 11 explains.

Your feet should be checked at every visit by your doctor, and twice a year by a foot specialist. If you have a serious problem with your feet, such as ingrown toenails or a fungal infection, your doctor should immediately refer you to a foot specialist, preferably one experienced in treating people with diabetes.

Foot problems require immediate attention because many people with diabetes have a lowered resistance to infections. People with diabetes often take between four to six weeks to heal after foot surgery, much longer than normal. For that reason, minor foot problems that should be treated promptly include ingrown or fungus toenails, athlete's foot, dry and cracked skin, calluses, ulcers, warts, foot deformities such as bunions and hammertoes, night cramps, and foot pain.

Charcot's foot occurs in approximately 1 in 700 people with diabetes. It appears most frequently in people who are overweight and who already have some loss of feeling, or neuropathy, in their feet. A Charcot break may occur in any bone in your foot or ankle. It occurs because the bones in the arch become soft; the arch can collapse, changing the weight-bearing dynamics of your foot. This can result in skin breakdowns or infections. If your foot unexplainably swells up with no break in the skin, and the foot feels unusually warm, these can be symptoms of a Charcot break. Charcot's foot is primarily treated by staying off your feet for several months, or by placing the foot in a cast.

When you have foot problems you should be referred to either a foot doctor, or *podiatrist,* or an *orthopedist,* who specializes in the foot and ankle. If your family doctor or primary care physician cannot refer you, your local medical association, American Diabetes Association, or professional groups such as the American College of Foot and Ankle Surgeons can help you.

Surgery can correct many foot deformities, such as hammertoes and bunions. Foot surgery is much more commonly done on people with diabetes now than in the past because a 1978 research study refuted the notion that blood vessels of people with diabetes collapse in the face of an infection, triggering gangrene. Vascular bypass surgery from the knee to the foot can be performed when an ulcer on the foot isn't healing and a greater blood supply is needed.

Exercises for people with foot problems: Any exercise program should minimize the stress on your feet. Exercises to help with peripheral neuropathy should lower blood sugar and increase strength, flexibility, and blood circulation. These include water aerobics, water sports, and swimming. Wear special water socks made of neoprene to protect the soles of your feet, since skin can be scratched on the bottom of a swimming pool. Never go barefoot. Some exercises may be done in a sitting position, as on a rowing machine. Bicycling, rowing, armchair exercises, and such floor exercises as leg lifts may be alternatives. Since muscles and joints may have lost flexibility, pain may be experienced. Take care that you don't overdo stretching exercises, since with neuropathy you've lost some feeling—you may sometimes lose warning signals of pain from the ligament areas. Don't put too much pressure on the joints by doing exercises such as deep knee bends. Check your feet before and after each exercise session as a matter of course.

EYE COMPLICATIONS

While blindness was once a common complication of diabetes, regular visits to eye specialists and good medical treatment have made it much less common, now affecting fewer than 2 percent of people with diabetes. Among older people with Type 2 diabetes, between 10 and 20 percent have some problem with their eyes, which weaken with age in all people. The eye does not require the presence of insulin to utilize glucose; many eye problems spring from the damage done by excess glucose to the tiny blood vessels in the eye. Approximately 90 percent of people with diabetes will have blood vessel changes in their eyes after having diabetes for twenty-five years.

Most eye complications are treatable. Laser treatment by *ophthalmologists,* or doctors specializing in the care of the eye, controls many eye problems by cauterizing the small blood vessels, but this must be coupled with effective blood sugar control to be successful. If eye complications are caught early enough, damage that has already occurred can sometimes be reversed.

The most serious eye complications are forms of *retinopathy,* the enlargement, breakage, or leaking of tiny blood vessels in the eye, which can spill blood into the eyeball to threaten vision.

Background retinopathy is a common complication of diabetes, involving tiny "bulges" that resemble miniature water balloons along the small eye vessels. Background retinopathy may be harmless. *Macular edema* is more serious; this occurs in the early stages of retinopathy, when retinopathy is concentrated on the small but crucial central part of the retina, called the *macula,* which controls daytime vision and color sensitivity. *Proliferative retinopathy* is a more advanced condition in which the bulges created during background retinopathy break and bleed onto the retina. This bleeding blocks vision and interferes with sight. Occasionally, the bleeding stops on its own, and the eye tissues merely absorb the blood. Proliferative retinopathy can be treated using the safe blue-green argon and green-only argon lasers, which are beams of light that cauterize broken blood vessels in the eye. This procedure can restore or improve sight, but it can also affect other aspects of sight such as peripheral vision and night vision.

A *vitreous hemorrhage* is a leaking of blood from vessels near the retina into the fluid inside the eyeball, which clouds the vision. A delicate surgical procedure called a *vitrectomy,* done in a hospital, can clear up this condition by removing the blood from inside the eye and replacing it with a clear fluid. This procedure can restore sight to people who have gone blind.

Cataracts cloud the lens of the eye, preventing light from entering. Cataracts are normally related more to aging than to diabetes, but poor blood sugar control can accelerate their development. If finances permit, artificial lenses may be implanted in the eye to replace lenses clouded over by cataracts.

Glaucoma, an eye disease in which pressure builds up inside the eye, occurs in older people, but is not directly related to diabetes. All people over age forty should be tested for glaucoma. Eyedrops can be prescribed to control it.

See an eye doctor immediately if you experience a sudden loss or change in vision, or if you have acute pain in your eye. Another symptom that needs immediate attention is the sensation of having a curtain lowered in the eyes. In these cases, insist that the eye doctor see you right away.

If your vision is impaired, the National Federation for the Blind, and the Braille Institute, whose telephone numbers are listed in the "Other Resources" appendix of this book, offer excellent programs to help people who are blind or partially sighted manage their day-to-day tasks. The National Federation for the Blind puts out an excellent free newspaper for people with diabetes, available in several forms including audiotape.

Exercises for people with eye complications: Cycling, swimming, or walking may be good aerobic exercises for people with retinopathy. Low-intensity exercises such as rowing machines, stationary bicycles, and treadmills also work well, as do some other exercise machines, tandem bicycling, and dancing. Exercises that jar the body or increase blood pressure, such as boxing, trampoline jumping, or weight lifting, should be avoided. Don't do exercises in which your head is lower than most of your body, such as handstands, diving, or such yoga postures as "the plow." Don't scuba dive or climb mountains, since the higher atmospheric or undersea air pressure poses additional risks to the eyes.

THE NERVES (NEUROPATHY)

Numbness in hands and feet, or cold, tingling, burning feelings can be symptoms of a common complication of the nerves or nervous system called *neuropathy*. Neuropathy typically begins with the so-called stocking and glove effect, which is a slight numbness that begins at the tips of the toes or fingers and then moves back. This is a problem because when you can't feel normal sensations such as pressure or pain, you can't compensate by shifting positions as you would otherwise. Neuropathy affects 60 to 70 percent of people with diabetes in mild to severe form. The pains associated with neuropathy frequently get worse at night, or during very hot or cold weather, and can be intensified by the touch of sheets or bedclothes. These feelings can last for months and then go away. They can also turn into numbness in the same areas caused by a blunted ability to feel sensations. Such numbness is a reason to inspect the feet and skin every day, and to always wear shoes when walking. It's best to not ignore these problems, because people with diabetes are twenty times as likely to experience nerve-related leg problems, such as gangrene and blockages, as will the general population.

Some types of neuropathy are manageable; the effects may sometimes be reversed by a combination of lowered blood sugar and medical treatment.

It is not fully understood why nerves are affected by diabetes. Nerves are somewhat like electric cords, with a protective outer layer of cells. One theory is that excess glucose in the blood may cause the outer *Schwann cells* that surround nerve bundles to swell, irritating and finally choking off the more functional inner nerve cells.

Sensory neuropathy is the form of neuropathy most closely associated with diabetes. One aspect of this, *peripheral neuropathy,* affects the areas of the body farthest from the heart, such as the legs, feet, arms, or hands, and sometimes the skeletal muscles. Numbness, coldness, or the feeling of walking on pins and needles can be symptoms. One effect of neuropathy is the common human experience of "foot drop," which occurs after you wake up and your foot feels like it's flapping when you walk. Neuropathy can manifest itself as a tight feeling in the chest, called *truncal neuropathy,* which is sometimes mistaken for a heart attack. Charcot's joint or a muscle-wasting condition called *amyotrophy* can result from sensory neuropathy. *Mononeuropathy* and *radiculopathy* are diseases of the spinal nerves or cranial nerves, which can sometimes be reversed.

Autonomic neuropathy involves the nerves whose functions are more or less automatic, nerves that control the stomach, sweat glands, digestive tract, intestinal system, bladder, penis, and circulatory system. *Gastroparesis,* a neuropathy-related digestive problem, can include symptoms of nausea, diarrhea, or constipation. Medications can give relief for most symptoms of gastroparesis, as can such simple changes in eating habits as eating smaller meals more frequently and adjusting the amount of fiber in your diet.

Good blood sugar control is the most effective single way to improve the symptoms of neuropathy, which may disappear over time. Mild pain relievers such as aspirin or Tylenol, or nonsteroidal, anti-inflammatory drugs, called NSAIDs, may be prescribed for pain. Antidepressant medications such as promazine or amitriptyline are sometimes prescribed in small amounts to help people with neuropathy. Drugs used to treat other disorders, such as the epilepsy drug gabapentin, sometimes bring relief. Local anesthetics and muscle relaxants also sometimes help. Narcotics such as codeine and morphine are almost never prescribed for neuropathy because they aren't particularly effective and can lead to drug dependence.

Folk remedies such as 2 teaspoons of apple cider vinegar with lunch can sometimes help mitigate night cramps, another manifestation of neuropathy. Cayenne pepper oil, applied topically while wearing gloves, sometimes relieves the "pins and needles" pain. The active ingredient in cayenne peppers, capsaicin, is the basis of over-the-counter medications such as Zostrix and ArthiCare, which are FDA approved for treating chronic pain, although they don't work for every person. Some people try Fosfree, a remedy available at health food stores. A quarter of a tablet of quinine sulfate is sometimes prescribed by doctors.

A study utilizing electrotherapy with Type 2 patients, reported in the spring 1999 issue of *Diabetes Technologies and Therapeutics*, showed that 83 percent of the patients whose lower extremities were treated for thirty minutes a day for a month reported relief. In a smaller substudy, two dozen patients found some additional pain relief by utilizing both electrotherapy and the antidepressant medication amitriptyline, 50 mg at bedtime. Transcutaneous electrical nerve stimulation (TENS) units use mild jolts of electricity and may be used at home, although they require a doctor's prescription.

A small study at New York Medical College completed in 1998 found that 75 percent of people with diabetic neuropathy who wore magnetic insoles in their shoes for four months had a reversal or reduction of their symptoms.

Self-help techniques that may help for foot neuropathy include soaking the feet for a few minutes in lukewarm water before bed. Walking around a bit before retiring can help. A foot cradle can be used to keep bedsheets from touching the feet at night. Stretching exercises may be helpful for muscle aches and pains.

In the realm of diet, some studies have also shown that increased doses of minerals and vitamins such as magnesium, calcium, and vitamin B6 (at a rate of 200 mg per day) can have a positive effect on neuropathy.

Stress-relieving techniques such as those listed in chapter 5 may help relieve some of the symptoms of neuropathy. Hypnosis, acupuncture, and massage may help to reduce stress or manage pain.

Exercises for people with peripheral neuropathy: If you have peripheral neuropathy, which affects balance and can numb the feet, avoid exercises that use the feet, such as jogging or running. Using a treadmill machine so that you can stabilize yourself is preferable. Swimming, water polo, aqua-aerobics, and exercises that can be done while seated are best. Bicycling, rowing, canoeing, floor exercises, and armchair exercises also work. To mitigate pain, stretch before doing exercise or yoga, but be careful to avoid overstretching the ligaments and muscles since you may not be able to feel certain pains. Check the feet for cuts or blisters before and after exercising, and wear good-fitting shoes and good clean socks.

Exercises for people with autonomic neuropathy: Since the autonomic nervous system controls sweating and other automatic functions, the ADA recommends that people with autonomic neuropathy avoid exercises that cause rapid changes in body position or that cause a sudden change in heart rate or blood pressure. Daily exercise is best, with slow and careful increases under a doctor's guidance. Adequate water should be consumed, and exercise in very hot or cold environments should be avoided.

KIDNEY AND URINARY TRACT COMPLICATIONS

The most serious complication of diabetes involving the urinary tract is *nephropathy,* which involves the kidneys. Nephropathy usually occurs in people who have had diabetes for a long time. It develops because the nephrons, or small arteries within the kidney, gradually harden. Nephropathy sometimes develops because of a urinary tract infection that has spread to the kidneys. According to one estimate, 20 to 30 percent of people with Type 2 diabetes may develop moderate to advanced kidney disease. Controlling your blood glucose levels and blood pressure will help prevent kidney disease, as will controlling cholesterol levels, stopping smoking, and perhaps consulting a dietitian to help you plan meals. If your doctor recommends it, some blood pressure medications such as ACE inhibitors can have a protective function for the kidneys.

Symptoms of nephropathy include swelling of the ankles, hands, face, or other body parts; loss of appetite, sometimes including a metallic taste in the mouth; skin irritations; difficulty thinking clearly; fatigue; or extreme difficulty managing blood sugar. Report any of these symptoms to the doctor who treats your diabetes.

In the least severe stages of kidney disease, called *microalbuminuria* and *proteinuria,* the kidneys release quantities of protein into the blood. *Uremia* results when the body retains waste products that are normally excreted. A swelling, called *edema,* occurs because excess fluid is retained in the body. Kidney and urinary tract complications may be treated by a kidney specialist, called a *nephrologist,* or by a *urologist,* who specializes in the care of the urinary tract.

Advanced kidney disease causes rising levels of the muscle waste product *creatinine. End-stage renal disease* occurs in approximately one-fourth of 1 percent of people with diabetes. It can be treated with *dialysis,* a process that periodically filters impurities from the blood. *Hemodialysis* takes blood out of the arm and runs it through a machine for three to five hours to filter out waste materials, then returns it to the body, a procedure done an average of three times a week. *Peritoneal dialysis* involves inserting a waste-absorbing fluid into the body through a tube inserted just below the navel; this can be done at home, several times a day. Peritoneal dialysis can also be done overnight, using a machine.

Kidney transplants can also be used to treat kidney failure. Transplanting one of the kidneys of a close relative versus an unrelated donor is generally preferred. Medical risks are involved in this operation since the immune system must be suppressed to allow the transplanted kidney to "take." Blood sugar control after the transplant is important.

According to Richard David, M.D., a Los Angeles urologist, 15 to 20 percent of people with diabetes who are over age sixty-five have some problem involving the urinary tract, kidneys, or bladder. Of these, up to 40 percent have trouble urinating, or have some bladder dysfunction. One reason for this is that excessive glucose in the bloodstream draws water out of the tissues, creating excessive urination, and neuropathy is another reason. Urological complications can often be prevented by good blood sugar control; if they develop, their progress can be stopped with good blood sugar control.

Symptoms of urinary tract infections include painful urination, frequent urination, and cloudy or bloody urine. In their earliest stages, urinary tract infections may have no symptoms at all, but show up on a urine test given by your doctor. As a general rule, bladder infections occur more frequently in people with diabetes. Infections of the urological tract, more common in women than in men, can begin in the bladder or ureters, and can sometimes spread to the kidneys, where they create additional problems. Kidney stones, for instance, can cause infections. Bladder infections may also be caused by incomplete emptying of the bladder; the infection often develops without painful symptoms, but it sometimes causes a bit of leakage. A *nonfunctioning bladder* may develop because of nerve damage in the bladder area associated with diabetes. When the bladder doesn't empty normally, urine is held longer and bacteria may grow. When blood sugars are elevated, sugar can be found in the urine. Bacteria multiply rapidly in a high blood sugar environment. Drinking plenty of water every day will help prevent a nonfunctioning bladder by flushing bacteria out of the system before they can multiply. Medications that you take can affect urination.

Most bladder infections can be successfully treated with bacteria-killing drugs called *antibiotics.* Your doctor may order a culture to determine which type of bacteria is causing your infection before writing a prescription—certain antibiotics are most effective on certain types of bacteria. If you are prescribed antibiotics, make sure that you take *all* the medicine prescribed for you, even if the symptoms subside while you still have medicine left. If you don't take all the medicine, you may miss killing a few of the stronger bacteria, and they will come back again, more resistant to antibiotics than before. This is true for all antibiotics.

Yeast infections in women flourish when blood sugar is high, so blood sugars should be controlled.

Neuropathy can also complicate bladder problems, since the blunted nerves don't always feel the bladder getting full. Neuropathy can cause you to lose the ability to squeeze the muscles that empty your bladder, resulting in *incontinence,* which strikes approximately 60 percent of people over sixty years of age whether or not they have diabetes. Incontinence may also be caused by weak abdominal muscles, muscle spasms in the bladder, or a blockage or other problem that prevents urination. Certain medications, irritating foods including alcohol and caffeine, impaired movement from arthritis or an injury, or poor blood sugar control can cause incidents of incontinence. Muscle-strengthening exercises, biofeedback, and drug and other medical treatments can help.

Even if you have begun to lose some kidney or urinary tract function, you can greatly slow down this process by maintaining good blood sugar control, and by modifying your diet, exercising, and taking medications as prescribed. Lowering your blood pressure slows kidney disease; you may be asked to take your blood pressure at home and report any changes to your doctor. Working with a registered dietitian or nutritionist to develop a proper diet, which may be low in sodium or protein, is a particularly important element in lowering blood pressure. Eliminating protein from animal sources is sometimes recommended. Medications can lower blood pressure and lighten the workload for the kidneys. Stress-reducing activities and exercise also help control blood sugar, as will full participation in the joyful events of your life.

Exercises for people with kidney problems: Don't exercise if you have excessive levels of protein in the urine, or *proteinuria*. Marathon running and long-distance bicycling in the heat should be avoided since they dehydrate the body and may cause more protein to accumulate in the urine. Avoid exercises that will increase blood pressure, such as weight lifting. Cycling, water exercises, archery, golf, and bowling may be fine. Moderate armchair-type exercises can be done almost any time, and will improve the patient's frame of mind as well as her ability to get around.

ISSUES SPECIFIC TO MEN

Impotence is a common complaint of men with diabetes. Between one-third and two-thirds of men with diabetes have trouble getting an erection. Impotence manifests itself as lessening rigidity of the penis, and the eventual inability to achieve an erection. This impotence is sometimes caused by nerve and small blood vessel damage, which is related to blood sugar control. Other male sexual problems related to diabetes can include retrograde ejaculation, in which ejaculation goes backward into the bladder, a condition that feels unusual but is not harmful. Retrograde ejaculation affects an estimated 2 percent of men who have diabetes.

Diabetic men have from two to five times the normal incidence of impotence, a condition that increases with age in the general population. Some men with diabetes may experience these problems ten to fifteen years earlier than normal. If your blood sugars are out of control, either too high or too low, bring them under control.

Impotence typically comes on gradually rather than suddenly appearing. If you are impotent with a sexual partner but continue to get erections in your sleep, your problem may be emotional or psychological. One method of determining this is to paste a strip of postage stamps onto your penis before you sleep. If the strip is broken in the morning, chances are you've had a nocturnal erection. If your doctor needs more precise information, *nocturnal tumescence monitoring* can be achieved by hooking yourself up to a machine for a night and letting the device record the number and intensity of your nighttime erections, according to Harley Wishner, M.D., a Los Angeles urologist.

Impotence is not always caused by diabetes. It can come from medications prescribed for other medical problems, such as high blood pressure, in which case discontinuing or changing medications may have a positive effect. The use of drugs such as tranquilizers, alcohol, or marijuana can cause impotence. Negative emotional stress affects the libido. Impotence frequently has psychological roots, even in men with diabetes, since even small decreases in potency can sometimes create an anxiety that further depresses sexual performance.

Men with diabetes who smoke run a greater risk of impotence. Since nicotine causes the blood vessels to constrict, smoking can reduce the supply of blood to the penis. A study of men conducted at Boston University Medical School found a decrease in blood flow to the penis in direct proportion to the number of cigarettes smoked. In Washington, D.C., a study of twenty impotent male smokers showed that seven of the twenty achieved nocturnal erections six weeks after they quit smoking.

If you are beginning to experience impotence, discuss this problem with your doctor. If you can do so, take your spouse or significant other to the doctor's office, and include her in some of the discussions. Your doctor may refer you to a urologist who specializes in the treatment of impotence, or to a mental health professional. If your impotence has a psychological or emotional basis, talking with a licensed therapist or a family therapist, or working with a sex counselor may help. A clinician trained in sex counseling may be found by contacting a professional organization such as the American Association of Sex Educators, Counselors, and Therapists, listed in the "Other Resources" appendix of this book.

If your doctor or urologist determines that your impotence has physical causes that cannot be corrected, several methods allow men to resume sexual activity, which is often connected to feelings of self-worth and self-esteem.

One such strategy involves the use of medicines called external vasodilators, ointments applied to the penis to stimulate blood flow. Although their effectiveness has not been scientifically proven, Minoxidil and nitroglycerine ointment may be useful when the problem involves insufficient blood flow through the arteries into the penis. Nitroglycerin ointment should be used with a condom, to prevent giving a sexual partner headaches after sex. Yohimbe, a folk remedy made from the bark of the yohimbe tree, may be useful in a few cases. Supplemental testosterone, a male hormone, may be administered by a doctor but it only increases potency if testosterone levels are abnormally low prior to treatment.

Among the drug treatments, the widely publicized sildenafil (Viagra) can help some men with diabetes. However, this drug has side effects that should be discussed with your doctor. Viagra should only be prescribed after a doctor's exam and the determination that your impotence has a chance of being treated by this means. Sildenafil can interact with drugs that expand the blood vessels such as nitroglycerin, and it is recommended that men stop those drugs for at least twenty-four hours before trying sildenafil. One study of men with diabetes found that men taking Viagra were successful in achieving suitable erections about half the time, versus about one-eighth of the time with a placebo. In research tests, sildenafil was most successful on men with milder impotence problems; that is, men who could achieve a partial but inadequate erection. Several similar drugs and a cream are currently in clinical trials.

An FDA-approved drug, sold under the brand name Caverject, has a success rate of about 80 percent. This drug may be injected into the base of the penis, causing an erection that lasts for a sufficient period of time. Drugs of this type are available with a doctor's prescription, but should be tested in the doctor's office prior to home use. These drugs have few side effects beyond the occasional scarring of the penis by the syringe, although some men experience pain where the drug is injected. An alternate method of administering a potency drug, the MUSE system, involves dispensing the medication directly into the urethra.

A commercial product sold under the brand name Rejoyn is a support sleeve that holds the flaccid penis in a rigid position to permit intercourse. Another commercial product is a vacuum cylinder device, which sells for about $200. These devices, which look a bit like bicycle tire pumps, create a vacuum that draws blood up into the penis to create an erection; a tension ring similar to a rubber band is placed at the base of the penis to hold the erection. The tension ring should be removed after half an hour to prevent bruising the penis.

The most expensive—and invasive—treatment involves prosthetic devices implanted in the penis. These devices have more than a 90 percent success rate. Surgery is involved, but the devices can be put to use almost immediately after you've healed from the surgery.

Keeping yourself healthy and controlling your blood sugar through stress reduction techniques, a balanced diet, and regular exercise is the best bet. And don't forget the other legitimate and pleasurable expressions of love. Beyond sexual intercourse, there are hundreds of ways to give yourself and your sexual partner mutual pleasure, including hugging, kissing, dancing, and sensual massage.

ISSUES SPECIFIC TO WOMEN

A study published in *The Journal of the American Medical Association* in 1999 found that 43 percent of women and 31 percent of men had a "sexual dysfunction," a term that includes not only impotence but also any trouble getting sexually aroused, loss of interest in sex, problems with orgasms, or other problems such as pain. Women with diabetes sometimes have sexual problems, including difficulty achieving sexual climax.

Women with diabetes sometimes complain of a loss of sensation in the genital region, which can inhibit sexual gratification. They are susceptible to yeast infections, which can make sexual intercourse painful. The normal volume of lubricating fluids produced in the vagina may diminish due to the effects of neuropathy, which may also be a cause of pain; both are related to blood sugar levels. Good blood sugar control is the only real cure for this condition, although your doctor may prescribe a salve to give some relief. The use of a safe, water-soluble vaginal lubricant such as K-Y Jelly, applied before intercourse, may be helpful in making intercourse more pleasurable for both partners.

Emotions such as fear, anxiety, resentment, and depression may inhibit sexual performance in women, as they can in men. If the roots of the problem are emotional, psychological or family counseling may help.

Women with Type 2 diabetes are fertile before menopause, and may become pregnant. Birth-control methods should be used until the pregnancy is wanted and can be planned. Women with diabetes should get their blood sugars under control before attempting to become pregnant, since poor blood sugar control is associated with birth defects, spontaneous abortions, and other complications. The subject of gestational diabetes, or diabetes that develops during pregnancy, is dealt with in chapter 12.

Estrogen therapy has its advantages and disadvantages. Glucose control and blood pressure are apparently not affected by estrogen replacement therapy. Women who take hormone replacement therapy after menopause have a 50 percent reduction in the chance of fatal heart attacks, a reduced incidence of bone loss, and perhaps slightly greater memory and brain function. However, the most significant risk for women is the possibility of a greater incidence of cancers such as breast cancer and endometrial cancer.

In general, women smokers are three times more likely to be infertile than are women nonsmokers, and they reach menopause two years earlier. Women who smoke are also more likely to have problems with pregnancy, and to have infants with birth defects.

SKIN PROBLEMS

Complications involving the skin are among the least serious complications of diabetes, but they can be troublesome and distressing because the skin involves everyone's self-image and self-esteem. The most visible skin problems are associated with poor control of blood sugars.

Xanthomas are orange fatty plaques that can appear around the eyes, on the elbows, on the shins, or on the ankles. They are sometimes related to fat levels in the body, particularly levels of cholesterol or triglycerides. Lowering the percentage of fat in your diet and achieving better blood sugar control can help make them go away. Doctors can prescribe medications to lower fat levels in the blood.

A physically disfiguring but medically harmless condition called *NLD,* or *necrobiosis lipoidica diabeticorum,* sometimes accompanies diabetes. NLD often appears as a pink or red discoloration, which tightens the skin and becomes shiny, not unlike the skin of a red apple. NLD is believed to develop when the skin gets thinner because of an inflammation, causing the loss of a normal layer of fat. NLD may first appear or intensify during times of poor blood sugar control. For some reason, NLD occurs more frequently in women than in men. Fortunately, it is completely harmless, and will eventually go away. No good treatment for NLD exists, although a few cases have responded to cortisone. Some clinical trials involving antiplatelet medications are underway to treat this condition by slowing its normal progress.

A yeast infection, *candidiasis,* can appear in the mouth, under the arms, or in the genital area, and may be treated with prescription medicines. If you develop many infections, boils, carbuncles, or other skin eruptions, your doctor may wish to take a culture and prescribe a medication to help clear them up. Additional insulin is sometimes prescribed.

So-called shin spots sometimes appear on the front of the legs, but they are harmless.

Since many skin problems are triggered or intensified by stress, using the stress-reduction techniques described in chapter 5 may help with control.

THYROID DISEASE

Thyroid disease is more common in people with Type 1 diabetes, but it sometimes develops in people with Type 2 diabetes. The thyroid is a small gland located in front of the windpipe that plays a role in metabolism.

People with diabetes have a 10 to 15 percent greater incidence of *hyperthyroidism,* in which an overactive thyroid gland secretes high levels of hormones, usually causing weight loss. Women over age forty, whether diabetic or not, are at increased risk. Both hyperthyroidism and *hypothyroidism,* in which an underactive gland causes weight gain, develop over a period of time and disturb efforts to control blood sugar.

Hashimoto's thyroiditis, an inflammation of the thyroid gland caused by an autoimmune attack, is the most common cause of thyroid disease.

Symptoms of thyroid disease include excessive nervousness, fatigue, or sleep problems. Thyroid problems should be treated by an *endocrinologist,* a doctor who specializes in the endocrine system, which includes the pancreas and the thyroid gland. A blood test called a *thyroid panel* is given when diabetes is diagnosed, or when thyroid problems are suspected.

HOSPITALIZATION

If you experience complications, or have other health problems not related to diabetes, you may find yourself in a hospital for a period of time. If you do land in the hospital, make sure that all your doctors and nurses understand that you have diabetes. Take all the precautions that you can.

If the hospital encourages it, and you have time to prepare for your stay, bring along your glucose meter and strips. Some hospitals encourage you to self-test, others require the use of their blood testing equipment. Bring your health insurance information. Bring your meal plan, the book in which you record your blood sugar levels, and any special equipment, vitamins, or clothes that you may need. Since the doctors whom you see in the hospital may need to know what medications you take, make a list that includes all of your medications, including insulin, and write down when you take each one. If you have time, you can make several copies of this list in advance, and give one to each person who asks for the information. It may make you feel more in control of the situation if you keep your own set of medical records while in the hospital, including a record of your test results.

If you don't understand the logic behind a treatment recommendation, buttonhole the appropriate doctor and ask questions. Have a spouse or a friend sit in on conferences with your doctors, if possible. You can also tape-record hospital discussions and listen to them later, when they might make more sense.

In most hospitals, you will probably have some help planning your meals. In states such as California, people with diabetes are legally required to have their nutritional needs assessed by a dietitian within seventy-two hours of entering a hospital. Dietitians often prescribe an ADA diet, but many hospitals provide a menu that allows you food choices. Some hospitals have a dietitian on staff, with whom you may be able to communicate.

If you feel up to it, ask your doctors for exercises to do while you're in the hospital. You may be able to remain physically active by doing armchair-type exercises in your hospital bed. If you're going to be in the hospital for several days, ask about the availability of physical therapy. Stress-relieving techniques such as deep breathing or visualization may be helpful. Most hospitals have chaplains who will speak with you when you ask for their services. Talking to a religious counselor could comfort you.

The American Hospital Association's Patient's Bill of Rights states that anytime you are hospitalized you have the right to receive complete information about your diagnosis, treatment, and expected outcome. You have the right to review your medical records, and to refuse any test or treatment. You have the right to keep the details of your treatment confidential from anyone not directly involved in your care—if you don't want a particular person to know the details of your medical condition, inform your caregivers of your wishes.

Keeping your blood sugar under control is important when you're hospitalized. If you are undergoing a physical stress such as surgery, your blood sugar levels will go up. Even if you don't normally take insulin, you may be given some to help you maintain control while being hospitalized.

Many of the medical complications of diabetes can be treated. The worst aspects of some complications may be mitigated by making a greater effort to control your blood sugars, and by adopting a program of good self-management that includes a well-balanced diet, exercise, and tests and treatments recommended by your medical team. Continue to learn, because new treatment methods can be quite effective. Your continuing role in self-management, the subject of the next chapter, remains the key to your empowerment and good health.

Chapter 16

NEW HORIZONS

Searching for the Cure for Diabetes

~

DIABETES IS A CHRONIC DISEASE THAT MUST BE MANAGED FOR THE REST OF YOUR LIFE. Although good self-management will help you control diabetes right now, medical breakthroughs could occur over the next few years to change how medical science thinks about this disease.

Receptionists at some chapters of the American Diabetes Association answer the telephone, "Until there's a cure." No one knows when that cure for diabetes may come, if it ever does. More than likely, progress in eradicating diabetes will be incremental, coming in thousands of small, painstaking steps rather than in one dramatic breakthrough such as the discovery of the first polio vaccine by Dr. Jonas Salk.

But every day, research continues, and it is realistic to expect that medical treatments will continue to improve. Continuing research into the effects of lifestyle changes, including the interaction of the mind with the body, as well as refinements in nutrition, pharmacology, and equipment technology may improve the lives of millions of people. For the present time, good self-management can hold diabetes at bay for a long time.

In the United States alone, about $12 billion a year is being spent on diabetes research. The National Institutes of Health, the American Diabetes Association, and the Juvenile Diabetes Foundation are the major sources of funding for this research. On the pharmacological front, promising new drugs being tested for the prevention or treatment of diabetic neuropathy include AGE inhibitors, neuroprotective drugs, antioxidant drugs, aldose-reductase inhibitors, and nerve growth factor. Alphareductase inhibitors are believed to prevent cataracts, and lipolic acid is being tested to see if it can prevent macular degeneration. Leptin, discovered with great hoopla in 1995 as a hormone linked to weight gain, is among the substances being tested as a weight-loss drug in humans.

All over the world, researchers are studying every conceivable aspect of diabetes treatment. An implantable insulin pump, developed by Medical Research Group LLC and already approved in the European community, is currently in the investigational stage at the FDA. Scientists are looking at particular combinations of stress-reduction techniques, nutritional strategies, and exercises. Transplants of real and artificial body parts are underway. Much research is going on at the cellular and molecular levels, quantifying the way in which various chemicals interact in the bodies of people with diabetes. Research scientists are looking at amylin, a hormone secreted from the pancreas (along with insulin), which is present insufficient amounts in people with diabetes. Amylin is being studied for its role in the metabolism of glucose, and analogues are being tested that may help make insulin replacement therapy more effective. According to an article in the May 7, 1999 *Los Angeles Times*, researchers have isolated a molecule from a fungus that controls blood glucose levels in diabetic mice. This molecule may be taken by mouth, raising the possibility it could have a similar effect in human beings, acting as a possible "insulin equivalent" that could replace injected insulin. The potential benefits of current research may only be imagined, since the results are as yet unknown.

PREVENTING DIABETES

Some current research focuses on identifying people with Type 2 diabetes at an earlier stage of their disease, or even before diabetes develops. Science may one day discover that diabetes is easier to prevent than to treat.

In 1996, the National Institute of Diabetes and Digestive and Kidney Diseases launched a long-term study called the Diabetes Prevention Program to identify whether four thousand overweight people over the age of twenty-five who have impaired glucose tolerance can prevent the onset of diabetes through dietary changes and exercise, or through preventive doses of diabetes drugs. Impaired glucose tolerance is an early indicator of Type 2 diabetes; each year another 7 percent of the 21 million Americans with this condition are diagnosed with Type 2 diabetes. The diabetes prevention trial is expected to be completed after the year 2000. At the University of Calgary in Alberta, Canada, a vaccine that prevents Type 1 diabetes with only one injection is currently being tested. An oral insulin has also been developed, and it is now being used in trials to see if it can prevent Type 1 diabetes. Scientists are examining the possibility that the presence of adequate levels of a simple B vitamin, niacin or nicotaminide, in residual cells may help prevent diabetes.

Genetic scientists are working to find the genes that identify a person likely to have Type 2 diabetes. The genetic connection has been established, since a history of first-degree relatives with Type 2 diabetes makes a diagnosis more likely within the family. A billion-dollar international scientific research effort, the Human Genome Project, is working to identify all the genes in the human body. The private sector is conducting genetics research for commercial purposes. Efforts are being made to identify the inherited gene and the chromosome that carry Type 2 diabetes.

When this gene or set of genes is identified, it may be possible for all people to be routinely tested for diabetes. If done on a large scale and followed by preventive measures, diabetes could be kept from developing in people predisposed to have it. It is theoretically possible to identify a gene that protects against diabetes and insert that gene into a living person such as a newborn baby. It is also theoretically possible, with the aid of genetic modifications, to produce insulin in other areas of the body. Better testing may one day help identify people at risk for particular complications, and create preventive treatments that mitigate the worst effects.

We already know that Type 2 diabetes can be slowed considerably by using many of the lifestyle changes recommended in this book. Since diabetes runs in families, you may be able to help your children and grandchildren by setting a good example and living a healthy lifestyle. You may want to share what you know, explaining how to reduce stress, enjoy healthy physical activity, and eat a healthy diet that helps control weight.

SCIENCE AND TECHNOLOGY

Transplants of the pancreas, the pancreas and kidneys, and the islet of Langerhans have met with some success for the past two decades. Several thousand of these transplants have been done, almost all on people with Type 1 diabetes, and only in a research setting. About one in four of these transplants fails.

Transplanting a body part from one person to another is extremely difficult. The recipient's immune system must be suppressed to prevent the body's natural tendency to reject something that is not of itself, even an organ such as a kidney that is needed for survival. Infection is also a major problem, since the immune system has already been suppressed by diabetes. Transplants of beta cells may be the most likely to succeed. One new technique utilizes the microencapsulation of beta cells into a membrane to protect these cells from the normal white blood cell immune response.

As equipment becomes more sophisticated, manufacturers make things smaller and lighter. Engineers are envisioning an artificial pancreas, somewhat like a pacemaker for the heart, that might be similar to timed-release birth-control pills and other medications that allow several months' supply to be implanted in the body. Insulin pumps may be the first step toward the development of a working artificial pancreas. A glucose sensor that works in tandem with the pump, which has already been approved for limited use, could be a second step. An artificial pancreas would mimic the normal operation of the human pancreas, continuously monitoring blood glucose levels, and releasing insulin as needed to keep blood sugar at a desirable level. A large machine called a Biostator can accomplish this already.

Innovations may come from computer technology, which can make rapid, complex, and precise mathematical calculations, and present the results in easily understood graphic form. A few computer software programs already contain glucose plotters, diet analyzers, and insulin therapy analyzers. When computer technology meets more sophisticated measuring and testing equipment, who knows the future possibilities for diet planning, insulin utilization, and blood glucose control? Infrared light beams, lasers, radio frequencies, and skin patches are now being used to develop the first noninvasive home blood testing equipment.

THE BEST RESPONSE

Until there's a cure, good self-management is the best response to diabetes. Find—and work with—good doctors, and a good health-care team. These people are your first line of defense. Educate yourself. Test your glucose as recommended, or whenever necessary. Take steps to relieve your stress. Eat regular, well-balanced meals that are appropriate for you. Remain physically active. Take the medications that your doctors prescribe. Don't ever stop educating yourself about ways to improve your health. If you continue to learn, you will continue to improve your self-management.

You will have difficult moments in your life whether or not you have diabetes. You will also have moments of pleasure and success. Participate in activities that you enjoy and that make your life worthwhile to you. Speak up for yourself when necessary. Communicate your feelings and thoughts to family and friends. Work to help other people as you can, and work to help yourself by maintaining a healthy social life.

Self-management is important. Practicing good self-management one day after the other will slowly but surely empower you.

OTHER RESOURCES

~

MANY EXCELLENT RESOURCES ARE AVAILABLE WHEN YOU'RE READY TO LEARN MORE about diabetes. This section includes contact information for government and nonprofit health organizations, educational organizations, professional groups, and some pharmaceutical companies and manufacturers. A short reading list of magazines and books follows, along with a few Internet and World Wide Web addresses.

I. GOVERNMENT, EDUCATIONAL, AND NONPROFIT ORGANIZATIONS

DIABETES INFORMATION

American Association of Diabetes Educators
100 W. Monroe, Chicago, IL 60603
This organization can provide a list of certified diabetes educators in your area. Telephone 1-800-338-3633 or (312) 424-2426
www.AADEnet.org

American Diabetes Association
1660 Duke Street, Alexandria, VA 22314
The largest diabetes organization in the world, encompassing professionals who treat people with diabetes. Makes recommendations on diabetes care, and publishes magazines, educational materials, and books. A source of information on clinical trials, local medical specialists, and support groups. Operators who speak English or Spanish will refer callers to state, provincial, or local associations that are good sources of information on local doctors, support groups, and other services.
Telephone 1-800-232-3472
www.diabetes.org

Canadian Diabetes Association
15 Toronto Street, Suite 800, Toronto, Ontario, Canada M5C2E3
Telephone (416) 363-0177

International Diabetes Center
3800 Park Nicollet Boulevard, St. Louis Park, MN 55416
Telephone (612) 993-3393

Joslin Diabetic Center
1 Joslin Place, Boston, MA 02215
A well-known diabetes care center, with several affiliates around the United States.
Telephone (617) 732-2415 or 1-800-567-5461

National Diabetes Education of the National Institutes of Health and the Centers for Disease Control and Prevention
One Diabetes Way, Bethesda, MD 20892-3600
This program offers two free educational kits for people with diabetes, "Feet Can Last a Lifetime" and "Do Your Level Best." Telephone 1-800-438-5383 or (301) 654-3327

National Diabetes Information Clearinghouse
1 Information Way, Bethesda, MD 20892
The National Institutes of Health's information clearinghouse on diabetes is a prime source of information. Telephone (301) 654-3327

National Kidney and Urologic Diseases Information Clearinghouse
3 Information Way, Bethesda, MD 20892-3580
Telephone (301) 654-4415

University of Michigan Media Library
2281 Bonisteel Boulevard, Ann Arbor, MI 48109
Telephone (734) 936-3191

MEDICAL INFORMATION

American Board of Medical Specialties
This organization will verify a doctor's credentials as a specialist,
or refer you to a board-certified specialist in your area.
Telephone 1-800-776-2378

American Board of Podiatric Surgery
This organization can provide a list of board-certified podiatrists in
your area. Telephone (415) 826-3200

American College of Foot and Ankle Surgeons
515 Busse Highway, Park Ridge, IL 60068-3150
Telephone 1-800-421-2237, (847) 292-2237, or 1-888-THE-FEET

Joint Commission on Accreditation of Healthcare Organizations
This organization checks and accredits hospitals in the U.S.
Telephone (603) 792-5000

The National Osteoporosis Foundation
1150 17th Street, Washington, DC 20036
Telephone 1-800-223-9994

The Neuropathy Association, Inc.
The Lincoln Building, 60 East 42 Street, Suite 942, New York, NY 10165
Telephone 1-800-247-6968
www.neuropathy.org

Visiting Nurse Association of America

11 Beacon Street, Suite 910, Boston, MA 02108

This organization can refer you to local organizations and nurses to provide home nursing services. Telephone 1-888-866-8773

ATHLETICS AND FITNESS

American College of Sports Medicine

PO Box 1440, Indianapolis, IN 46206

Telephone (317) 637-9200

American Council on Exercise

5820 Oberlin Drive, No. 102, San Diego, CA 92121

Telephone 1-800-825-3636 or (619) 535-8227

For information on walking or hiking clubs in a particular area, contact:

American Volks-Sports Association

1001 Pat Boorer Road, Universal City, TX 78148

Telephone (210) 659-2112

Aquatic Exercise Association

PO Box 1609, Nokomis, FL 34274

Telephone (941) 486-8600

Armchair Fitness Videos focus on strength improvement, stretching, aerobics, gentle exercise, yoga, and other topics for people who must limit vigorous activity. They are available from:

CC-M, Inc.

8510 Cedar Street, Silver Spring, MD 20910

Telephone 1-800-453-6280

International Diabetic Athletes Association

1647 West Bethany Home Road, Suite B, Phoenix, AZ 85015

This organization is a networking clearinghouse for people interested in the special relationship between exercise enthusiasts and diabetes, and

for health-care professionals interested in diabetes and sports.
Telephone 1-800-898-4322 or (602) 433-2113

National Organization of Mall Walkers
PO Box 256, Hermann, MO 65041
Telephone (573) 486-3945

Sierra Club
85 Second Street, San Francisco, CA 94105
The Sierra Club has chapters all over the U.S. that organize hiking,
trekking, backpacking, and other outdoor athletic activities.
Telephone (415) 977-5500

United States Blind Athletes Association
33 North Institute Street, West Hall, Colorado Springs, CO 80903
Telephone (719) 630-0422

YMCA of the USA
Telephone 1-800-872-9622

ACUPUNCTURE

American Academy of Medical Acupuncture
5820 Wilshire Boulevard, No. 500, Los Angeles, CA 90036
This organization can recommend a doctor who practices acupuncture.
Telephone 1-800-521-2262 or (323) 937-5514

BIOFEEDBACK

To locate a clinician skilled in biofeedback, contact:

Association for Applied Psychophysiology and Biofeedback
10200 W. 44th Avenue, No. 304, Wheat Ridge, CO 80033
Telephone (303) 422-8436

DIET

American Dietetic Association
216 West Jackson Boulevard, No. 800, Chicago, IL 60606
This organization will provide a list of registered dietitians in your area.
Telephone 1-800-366-1655 or 1-800-877-1600
www.eatright.org

Weight Watchers
175 Crossways Park West, Woodbury, NY 11797
Telephone 1-800-651-6000

Overeaters Anonymous
PO Box 44020, Rio Rancho, NM 87174-4020
Telephone (505) 891-1664

FINANCIAL AND INSURANCE INFORMATION

Medicare Information Line provides information about Medicare, Medicare supplemental insurance, HMOs, and special programs for low-income people. Telephone 1-800-638-6833

For financial help with some ancillary costs not covered by Medicare for dialysis and kidney transplants, some assistance may be available through:

National Kidney Foundation
30 E. 33 Street, New York, NY 10016
Telephone 1-800-622-9010

American Kidney Fund
6110 Executive Boulevard, Suite 1010, Rockville, MD 20852
Telephone 1-800-638-8299 or (301) 881-3052

Pharmaceutical Research and Manufacturers of America
1100 15th Street, NW, Washington, DC 20005
This group will provide a brochure listing the programs offered by drug companies to help people without insurance secure necessary medicines.

Telephone 1-800-762-4636 or (202) 835-3400
www.phrma.org/patients

President's Committee on Employment of People with Disabilities
This organization provides information on the Americans with Disabilities
Act. Telephone (202) 376-6200

U.S. Equal Opportunity Commission
Telephone 1-800-792-5259

American Association of Retired Persons (AARP)
601 E Street NW, Washington, DC 20049
Telephone 1-800-441-2277
www.aarp.org

SEX THERAPY

American Association of Sex Educators, Counselors, and Therapists
PO Box 238, Mt. Vernon, IA 52314-0238
This is a professional organization that can refer you to a practitioner of
sexual therapy in your area. Telephone (319) 895-8407, fax (319) 895-6203,
or e-mail AASECT@worldnet.att.net

American Association for Marriage and Family Therapy
www.aamft.org/faqs/DirPub.htm

Impotence Institute of America
PO Box 410, Bowie, MD 20718-0410
Telephone 1-800-669-1603
www.impotenceworld.org

SIGHT IMPAIRMENT

American Council for the Blind
1155 15th Street, NW, Washington, DC 20005
Telephone 1-800-424-8666

Braille Institute

741 N. Vermont Avenue, Los Angeles, CA 90029

The Braille Institute offers classes in several California cities on survival skills, measuring and injecting insulin, cooking, and other skills for blind and partially sighted people. Telephone 1-800-272-4553 or (323) 295-4050

Guide Dogs for the Blind

Telephone 1-800-295-4050

www.guidedogs.com

The National Federation of the Blind

1800 Johnson Street, Baltimore, MD 21230

The Diabetes Action Network produces an excellent free newsletter, *Voice of the Diabetic,* available in print or audio cassette. The federation offers classes and educational programs, some several months long, which focus on living skills and coping with blindness.

Telephone (410) 659-9314.

www.nfb.org

U.S. Library of Congress

Talking books and disks.

Telephone (202) 707-5000

STOP SMOKING

American Heart Association offers a free stop-smoking kit called "Calling It Quits." Telephone 1-800-242-8721

www.americanheart.org

American Lung Association offers stop-smoking information.

Telephone 1-800-586-4872

SUPPORT GROUPS

American Diabetes Association will refer you to a local support group.

Telephone 1-800-232-3472

Friends Health Connection

PO Box 114, New Brunswick, NJ 08903
This organization connects people with similar health problems.
Telephone 1-800-48-FRIEND.
www.48friend.com

National Family Caregivers Association

10605 Concord Street, Suite 501, Kensington, MD 20895-2504
This is a nonprofit organization that provides networking services for
caregivers of all types. Telephone 1-800-896-3650
www.nfcacares.org

TRAVEL

Diabetes Traveler

PO Box 8223 RW, Stamford, CT 06905
This is a newsletter specializing in information for people with
diabetes who travel.
Telephone (203) 327-5832
www.ishops.com/diabetes

International Diabetes Federation

International Association Center, 40 Washington Street, B-1050, Brussels,
Belgium 32-2-647 44 14
This federation sponsors World Diabetes Day, and can provide a list of
doctors who specialize in treating diabetes for foreign travelers.
www.idf.org

International Association of Medical Assistance for Travellers

417 Center Street, Lewiston, NY 14092
This association publishes and sells a directory of English-speaking doctors around the world. Telephone (716) 754-4883

YOGA

International Association of Yoga Therapists
20 Sunnyside Avenue, Suite A-243, Mill Valley, CA 94941
Telephone (415) 332-2478

II. PHARMACEUTICAL AND EQUIPMENT COMPANIES

GLUCOSE METER MANUFACTURERS

LifeScan, a Johnson & Johnson company
1000 Gibraltar Drive, Milpitas, CA 95035-6312
Telephone 1-800-227-8862 (twenty-four hour line)
www.lifescan.com

Roche Diagnostics Corporation
9115 Hague Road, PO Box 50100, Indianapolis, IN 46256
Telephone 1-800-858-8072
www.roche.com

Bayer, Diagnostics Division
c/o Bayer Corporation, 511 Benedict Avenue, Tarrytown, NY 10591
Telephone 1-800-348-8100
www.bayerdiag.com

Medisense, Inc.
4A Crosby Drive, Bedford, MA 01730
Telephone 1-800-527-3339
www.abbott.com

Cascade Medical
10180 Viking Drive, Eden Prairie, MN 55344
Telephone 1-800-525-6718

INSULIN PUMPS

Disetronic Medical Systems, Inc.
5201 East River Road, No. 312, Minneapolis, MN 55421-1014
Telephone 1-800-280-7801
www.disetronic.com

MiniMed Technologies
12744 San Fernando Road, Sylmar, CA 91342
Telephone 1-800-933-3322
www.minimed.com

INSULIN MANUFACTURERS

Eli Lilly Company
Lilly Corporate Center, Indianapolis, IN 46285
Telephone 1-800-545-5979 or (317) 276-2000
www.lilly.com

Novo-Nordisk Pharmaceuticals, Inc.
100 Overlook Center, Suite 200, Princeton, NJ 08540
Telephone 1-800-727-6500
www.novo-nordisk.com

MEDICAL SUPPLIES

Diabetic.com
3275 W. Hillsboro Boulevard, Suite 201, Deerfield Beach, FL 33442
Telephone 1-800-342-2384
www.diabetic.com

Medic Alert Foundation International
2323 Colorado Avenue
Turlock, CA 95382
Telephone 1-800-432-5378

Maxi-Aids
42 Executive Boulevard, Farmingdale, NY 11735
This company sells products for people with visual and physical impairments. Telephone 1-800-522-6294

III. OTHER READING

MAGAZINES AND NEWSLETTERS OF INTEREST

Diabetes Forecast
Published by the American Diabetes Association, 1660 Duke Street, Alexandria, VA 22314
A monthly magazine that publishes an annual buyer's guide to diabetes products. Telephone 1-800-232-3472

Diabetes Self-Management
R.A. Rappaport Publishing, 150 W. 22nd Street, New York, NY 10011
A monthly magazine. Telephone 1-800-234-0923

Diabetes Interview
3715 Balboa Street, San Francisco, CA 94123
Telephone 1-800-234-1218 or (415) 387-4002

Practical Diabetes International
PMH Publications, Box 100, Chichester, West Sussex, PO18 8HD, United Kingdom

SOME BOOKS OF INTEREST

Anderson, James, M.D. *Diabetes: A Practical New Guide to Healthy Living.* New York: Warner Books, 1991.

Beaser, Richard S., M.D., and Joan V.C. Hill, R.D., C.D.E. *The Joslin Guide to Diabetes: A Program for Managing Your Treatment.* New York: Simon & Schuster, 1995.

Bernstein, Richard D., M.D. *Diabetes Type II: Including Dramatic New Approaches to the Treatment of Type 1 Diabetes.* Englewood Cliffs, N.J.: Prentice-Hall Press, 1990.

Cousins, Norman. *The Healing Heart.* New York: W.W. Norton, 1983.

Edelwich, Jerry, and Archie Brodsky. *Diabetes: Caring for Your Emotions.* New York: Addison-Wesley, 1986.

Ezrin, Calvin, M.D., and Robert E. Kowalski. *The Type II Diabetes Diet Book.* Los Angeles: Lowell House, 1995.

Gordon, Neil F., M.D., Ph.D., M.P.H. *Diabetes: Your Complete Exercise Guide.* Champaign, Ill.: Human Kinetics, 1993.

Graham, Claudia, C.D.E., Ph.D., M.P.H., June Biermann, and Barbara Toohey. *The Diabetes Sports and Exercise Book.* Los Angeles: Lowell House, 1995.

Guthrie, Diana W., R.N., Ph.D., and Richard A. Guthrie, M.D. *The Diabetes Sourcebook: Today's Methods and Ways to Give Yourself the Best Care, 4th ed.* Los Angeles: Lowell House, 1999.

Hansen, Barbara Caleen, Ph.D., and Shauna S. Roberts, Ph.D. *The Commonsense Guide to Weight Loss for People with Diabetes.* Alexandria, Va.: Amercian Diabetes Association, 1998.

Jovanovic-Peterson, Lois, M.D., Charles M. Peterson, M.D., and Morton B. Stone. *A Touch of Diabetes: A Straightforward Guide for People Who Have Type II, Non-Insulin-Dependent Diabetes.* Minneapolis: Chronimed Publishing, 1995.

Lodewick, Peter A., M.D. *A Diabetic Doctor Looks at Diabetes: His and Yours.* Los Angeles: Lowell House, 1998

Monk, Arlene, R.D., C.D.E., et al. *Managing Type II Diabetes.* Wayzata, Minn.: DCI Publishing, 1988.

Ornish, Dean, M.D. *Dr. Dean Ornish's Program for Reversing Heart Disease.* New York: Ballantine Books, 1990.

Peterson, Charles M., M.D., and Lois Jovanovic, M.D. *The Diabetes Self-Care Method, 3d ed.* Los Angeles: Lowell House, 1998.

Rosenthal, M. Sara. *The Type 2 Diabetic Woman.* Los Angeles: Lowell House, 1999.

Walsh, John, P.A., C.D.E., and Ruth Roberts. *Pumping Insulin: Everything in a Book for Successful Use of an Insulin Pump.* San Diego, Calif.: Torrey Pines Press, 1994.

SOME COOKBOOKS OF INTEREST

American Diabetes Association Month of Meals, a Menu Planner. American Diabetes Association, 1660 Duke Street, Alexandria, VA 22314. Published 1989.

Brody, Jane. *Jane Brody's Good Food Book.* New York: Bantam, 1987.

Cooper, Nancy. *The Joy of Snacks.* Minneapolis: Chronimed, 1991.

Exchange Lists and Meal Planning. American Diabetes Association and American Dietetic Association, revised 1995. Available in braille and on audio cassette from American Diabetes Association, 1660 Duke Street, Alexandria, VA 22314.

Family Cookbooks, Volumes I, II, III, and IV. A collaboration between the American Diabetes Association and American Dietetic Association, 1660 Duke Street, Alexandria, VA 22314.

The Fat Counter. New York: Pocket Books, 1993.

Finsand, Mary Jane. *The Complete Diabetic Cookbook.* New York: Sterling Publishing Company, 1987.

Gillard, Judy, and Joy Kirkpatric. *The Guiltless Gourmet.* Nutrition Wise Partnership, PO Box 499, Rancho Mirage, CA. Published 1990.

Marks, Betty. *Microwave Diabetic Cookbook.* Chicago: Surrey Books, 1991.

Nissenberg, Sandra K., M.S., R.D., Margaret L. Bogle, Ph.D., R.D., and Audrey Wright, M.S., R.D. *Quick Meals for Healthy Kids and Busy Parents*. Minneapolis: Chronimed Publishing, 1995.

Polin, Bonnie, Fran Giedt, and Joslin Nutrition Services Department. *The Joslin Diabetes Gourmet Cookbook*. New York: Bantam Books, 1994.

Soneral, Lois. *The Type II Diabetes Cookbook*. Los Angeles: Lowell House, 1997.

Soneral, Lois M. *The Type 2 Diabetes Desserts Cookbook*. Los Angeles: Lowell House, 2000.

Warshaw, Hope S., R.D., C.D.E. *The Restaurant Companion*. Chicago: Surrey Books, 1990.

Wedman, Betty. *American Diabetes Association Holiday Cookbook*. Englewood Cliffs, N.J.: Prentice-Hall, 1986.

IV. ELECTRONIC INFORMATION

Personal computer users can access medical information via the Internet, and many sites contain useful information. In addition to the brief sampling of sites listed here, all the major commercial on-line services, such as Compuserve and America Online, have forums and newsgroups where diabetes is discussed. A caveat: not everything posted on-line is true. Use the same caution about statements you read electronically as you would if you heard a statement about diabetes from a stranger, even one who claims to have medical credentials. Information posted on university and government medical databases is typically reliable and up-to-date, as is information posted by major nonprofit health organizations such as the American Diabetes Association.

A FEW WORLD WIDE WEB SITES

www.niddk.nih.gov
The federal government's National Institutes of Health, National Institute of Diabetes and Digestive and Kidney Diseases Web page contains a good overview of diabetes, a glossary of terms related to diabetes, relevant statistics, and contact information on professional and voluntary diabetes organizations. Also, here is the latest information on the Diabetes Control and Complications Trial. Visitors can jump from here to other NIH Web sites.

www.diabetes.org
American Diabetes Association home page.

www.biostat.wisc.edu/diaknow;index.htm
Diabetes Knowledgebase at the University of Wisconsin aims to be a comprehensive educational resource for people with diabetes and health-care professionals. Provides links to other sites of interest, lists frequently asked questions about diabetes, and provides information on groups for people with diabetes. Includes the Diabetic Friends Action Network newsletter, a glossary, and a glycemic index page.

www.lehigh.edu/lists/diabetic
LeHigh Diabetic Archives contain answers to the most frequently asked questions (FAQs) about diabetes from queries to its mailing list.

www.cdc.gov/nccdphp/ddt/dthome.htm
Federal Center for Disease Control's diabetes page.

www.eatright.org
American Dietetic Association home page.

www.diabetesnet.com/index.html
Diabetes Net is one of the sites that features commercial products and related information for the person with diabetes.

www.ummed.edu/dept/diabetes
Healing Handbook for Persons with Diabetes, by University of Massachussetts Medical Center.

www.cookinglight.com
Cooking Light magazine Web site includes recipes and nutritional information.

www.onhealth.com
Published in association with the International Diabetes Center. Has information on treatments, self-management, and lab tests. Provides on-line discussion groups. Also has recipes.

www.gourmetconnection.com
Diabetes Gourmet magazine. Great recipes and information.

www.diabetesnet.com
Diabetes Mall. Information, links to other diabetes sites, how to e-mail politicians, an on-line store for diabetic products, and an on-line newsletter, *Diabetes This Week*.

www.joslin.org
The site for the Joslin Diabetes Center at Harvard Medical School. Up-to-the-minute news stories on diabetes; research information; loads of educational material with an on-line diabetes library, catalog of publications, and discussion groups.

www.intelihealth.com
Intelihealth, the Johns Hopkins Hospital Health Information site. Provides extensive information plus a drug search site.

www.centerwatch.com
Center Watch: clinical trials listings.

www.ndei.org
National Diabetes Education Initiative (Type 2).

www.diabeteswell.com
Diabetes Well.

www.mdcc.com
Diabetes Monitor

A FEW ADDITIONAL INTERNET SITES OF INTEREST

misc.health.diabetes
A forum where the everyday issues involving the management of diabetes are discussed, including medical breakthroughs, diet, exercise, blood glucose control, and relevant activities.

listserve@netcom.com
A free weekly newsletter, *The Diabetes Interview Newsletter,* may be obtained if you send to the above address and write: subscribe diabetes-news.

alt.support.diabetes.kids
A forum for parents and caregivers of children with diabetes.

idaa@getnet.com
International Diabetic Athletes Association

GLOSSARY OF COMMON TERMS

~

ACIDOSIS A medical condition that can occur in people not producing insulin in their bodies, or who do not receive adequate insulin, causing the body to become acidic.

ADULT ONSET DIABETES Non-insulin-dependent diabetes mellitus, or Type 2 diabetes. A term once commonly used for Type 2 diabetes.

ATHEROSCLEROSIS A disease in which fat accumulates in blood vessels, which can slow down or stop blood flow.

BETA CELLS Cells located in the pancreas, which produce insulin.

BLOOD GLUCOSE LEVEL A form of digested sugar, called glucose, in the bloodstream is commonly known as "blood sugar." The blood glucose level is the concentration of glucose in the blood at a particular time. In the United States, this is measured in milligrams per deciliter or mg/dl. Some countries measure this in millimols per liter or mmol/L.

BLOOD SUGAR TEST A simple medical test in which a person with diabetes uses a blood glucose meter to check the level of glucose in his or her blood.

CALORIE A measure of food energy. Technically, a calorie is the amount of energy needed to raise the temperature of a thousand grams of water 1 degree centigrade.

CARBOHYDRATE A primary and necessary category of nutrients for the body, composed mainly of starches and sugars.

CARDIOVASCULAR DISEASE A disease of the heart and large blood vessels that can occur more frequently in people with diabetes.

CERTIFIED DIABETES EDUCATOR A diabetes educator who has passed a comprehensive test on the management of diabetes given by the National Certification Board for Diabetes Educators.

CHARCOT'S BREAK A degeneration of the stress-bearing action of joints, such as the ankles, which is chronic and progressive.

CHOLESTEROL A fatlike substance, necessary for good health, which is manufactured in the body, and which can be eaten in foods. Can increase the risk for heart disease when levels are too high.

COMBINATION THERAPY Treatment utilizing more than one medication.

COMPLICATIONS OF DIABETES Medical complications of diabetes can involve the feet, eyes, nerves, teeth, cardiovascular system, skin, thyroid gland, kidneys, and urinary tract.

DAWN PHENOMENON A typical rise in blood sugar levels in the early morning.

DIABETOLOGIST A medical doctor specializing in the treatment of diabetes.

DIETITIAN A person who helps plan meals for people with special health needs. A *registered dietitian* is one who has been certified as a specialist in this area by the American Dietetic Association.

EMPOWERMENT A name for the process by which an individual gains a measure of power and control over his or her own life.

ENDOCRINOLOGIST A medical doctor who treats problems relating to the endocrine system, including the hormone-producing glands of the body, such as the pancreas and thyroid glands.

EXERCISE PHYSIOLOGIST A medical specialist who understands how physical activity affects the cells, tissues, and organs of the human body.

FAT A nutrient needed to sustain life, as in saturated and unsaturated fats.

GESTATIONAL DIABETES Diabetes that appears for the first time during pregnancy, and which should be treated. Can sometimes be a precursor of Type 2 diabetes.

GLUCAGON A hormone manufactured in the pancreas that raises the level of sugar in the blood, complimenting the action of another hormone, insulin, which lowers blood sugar.

GLUCOSE A medical term for a form of sugar found in the blood that is used by the body's tissues for energy.

GLUCOSE TOLERANCE TEST A medical test, sometimes called the oral glucose tolerance test, or OGTT, in which the patient drinks a particular amount of glucose, and then has blood glucose levels measured for periods of time after ingestion. Used to diagnose gestational diabetes.

GLYCEMIC CONTROL A medical term for controlling blood sugar levels. Also called blood glucose control.

GLYCOGEN The form in which glucose is stored in the liver, after conversion by a natural process called *glycogenesis*. Glycogen can be released back into the bloodstream as glucose during a fast or during an insulin reaction.

GLYCOSYLATED HEMOGLOBIN TEST or **HbA1C TEST** Nearly identical blood tests that measure the average blood sugar level during the past few months. Used by a doctor to get a quick read on how a particular patient is managing his or her blood sugar levels.

GRAM A tiny metric unit of weight used to determine how much of which foods to eat during dieting. There are 453 grams in 1 pound.

HDL CHOLESTEROL The "good" high-density lipoprotein cholesterol, the form in which cholesterol is swept from the body.

HEMOGLOBIN A1 and **HEMOGLOBIN A1c** Protein substances in the red blood cells that carry oxygen to body tissues. Measurement of the level of blood sugar attached to these proteins is done in a glycosylated hemoglobin test.

HIGH BLOOD SUGAR Excessive blood glucose levels. Also called hyperglycemia.

HORMONE A chemical produced in a gland or tissue of the body that stimulates an effect in other tissues or organs after being carried there in the bloodstream. Insulin and adrenalin are hormones.

HYPERGLYCEMIA A medical term for high blood sugar.

HYPERTENSION A medical term for high blood pressure.

HYPERTROPHY A medical term for thick, puffy skin over the site where insulin is injected, which may slow down the rate of absorption of insulin in people who inject it.

HYPOGLYCEMIA A medical term for low blood sugar.

HYPOGLYCEMIC AGENT A drug that can lower blood sugar levels.

INJECTION AREAS Areas on the body into which insulin can be injected, such as the abdomen, the outer area of the upper arm, the upper area of the buttocks, and the outer front of the middle of the thigh. The location of each injection given is called an *injection site*.

INSULIN A chemical hormone manufactured in the pancreas and released into the bloodstream, which lowers the sugar level in the blood by helping the body tissues utilize digested food.

INSULIN REACTION Symptoms experienced by people with very low blood sugar, including weakness, shakiness, nervousness, sweatiness, or confusion.

ISLETS OF LANGERHANS The part of the pancreas gland that produces insulin and glucagon.

KETOACIDOSIS A serious medical condition combining ketosis and acidosis. When inadequate insulin exists in the body, large amounts of sugar and ketones accumulate in the blood and urine. Affects people with Type 1 diabetes, not Type 2.

KETONES Chemicals produced when the body burns fat for energy, rather than sugar.

KETOSIS A potentially serious medical situation in which ketones are present in the urine due to excessive breakdown of fats.

KIMMELSTIEL-WILSON SYNDROME A medical term, first described by two doctors, for lesions on the kidneys that are caused by a degeneration of the blood vessels as a result of diabetes that is poorly controlled.

LDL CHOLESTEROL Low-density lipoprotein cholesterol or "bad" cholesterol is the form of cholesterol that remains in the blood. High levels of LDL cholesterol increase the risk of heart disease.

LIPID A scientific name for fats in the body.

LOW BLOOD SUGAR Blood glucose levels that are excessively low. Also called hypoglycemia.

MAINTENANCE DOSE The dose of a particular drug that achieves stability for a period of time.

MEAL PLAN A strategy for eating carefully, in which particular foods are chosen to be eaten at particular times and in particular amounts.

MENTAL HEALTH PROFESSIONAL A person who specializes in mental health, who may counsel individuals during times of great emotional need. Can be a psychiatrist, who is a medical doctor specializing in mental health and who can prescribe medications. May also be a psychologist or social worker. May work with either individuals or groups with particular needs.

METABOLISM A medical term for the ongoing chemical processes inside the body, such as those that convert food into energy, which collectively keep the body alive.

MG/DL Milligrams per deciliter. Used to measure blood sugar and levels of some other chemicals in the body.

MICROALBUMINURIA An early sign of kidney disease in which small amounts of protein are detected in the urine.

MICROANEURYSMS In the very small blood vessels called capillaries, such as those found on the retina of the eye, these are small opened-out areas that can burst or bleed.

MONOTHERAPY Treating a disease with one drug rather than several.

NEPHROPATHY A medical term for kidney damage occurring in the filtering portions, or *nephrons,* of the kidneys, which may occur as a long-term effect of diabetes.

NEUROPATHY Nerve tissue damage that may occur as a long-term complication of diabetes.

NON-INSULIN-DEPENDENT DIABETES MELLITUS Another name for Type 2, or adult onset, diabetes. Abbreviated NIDDM.

NUTRITIONIST A person who provides advice on nutrition.

OPHTHALMOLOGIST A medical doctor specializing in the care of the eyes.

ORAL HYPOGLYCEMIC AGENT A pill that lowers blood sugar.

ORTHOPEDIST A medical doctor who deals with the locomotor structures of the body, such as the bones, joints, and muscles. Can specialize in particular areas, such as the feet and ankles.

PANCREAS An organ just behind the stomach that produces insulin, glucagon, and digestive enzymes.

PANCREAS (ARTIFICIAL) A small machine that withdraws and reinserts blood into the body, mimicking the functions of the beta cells. It can be set to inject insulin or glucose to maintain normal levels in the blood.

PODIATRIST A doctor specializing in the care of feet.

POLYDIPSIA A medical term for extreme thirst that comes with increased drinking of water.

POLYPHAGIA A medical term for excessive hunger resulting in more eating.

POLYURIA A medical term for excessive output of urine.

PREMIXED INSULIN   An insulin containing a mixture of short- and intermediate-acting insulins, such as 70/30.

PROTEIN   A nutrient required to sustain life, used to build and repair body tissues.

RECOMBINANT DNA TECHNOLOGY   The chemical process of making biosynthetic human insulin.

RENAL   A medical term for something having to do with the human kidneys.

RENAL THRESHOLD   The so-called spill point, a bit different in every person, at which glucose is drawn out of the bloodstream and begins to spill from the kidneys into the urine.

RETINOPATHY   A medical term for damage to the eye, specifically the blood vessels of the retina at the back of the eye, which can be a long-term complication of diabetes. Includes *background* retinopathy, and the more advanced *proliferative* retinopathy, which cause blurred vision and other symptoms.

SATURATED FAT   A type of fat, usually derived from animal sources, that is solid at room temperature. Lard and butter are examples of foods that contain saturated fats.

SELF-MANAGEMENT   All your efforts to control diabetes, which may include stress reduction, blood glucose testing, dietary changes, exercise, and the use of medications.

SELF-MONITORING   Your own testing and recording of test results, such as blood glucose or sugar levels.

SULFONYLUREA   A class of drugs that stimulate the pancreas to produce additional insulin.

SUPPORT GROUP A group of people, and sometimes family members, who share a common disease or concern, who meet on a regular basis to discuss life issues, often with a trained group leader.

TYPE 1 DIABETES Once known as juvenile onset diabetes, a type of diabetes in which the body does not manufacture insulin. Also known as insulin dependent diabetes mellitus or IDDM.

TYPE 2 DIABETES Once known as adult onset diabetes, a type of diabetes most commonly found in older adults. The most common type of diabetes, Type 2 diabetes is a condition in which insulin is available to the body but it cannot be properly utilized. Also called non-insulin-dependent diabetes mellitus or NIDDM, non-ketosis-prone diabetes, adult diabetes, or maturity-onset diabetes in the young (MODY).

UNSATURATED FATS Fats that are typically liquid at room temperature, such as vegetable oils. *Monounsaturated fats* such as those in foods such as olive oil, do not lower HDL cholesterol. *Polyunsaturated* fats, such as those in foods such as corn oil, are more chemically complex forms of unsaturated fats.

INDEX

~

A

Y

Z